EMERGENCY
FIRST AID
FOR DOGS

SHELDON RUBIN, DVM
edited by W. I. ATKINSON, BVMS, MRCVS

Frederick Muller Limited
London SW19 7JU

This publication is not to be used in place of a veterinary surgeon, but merely to guide you in helping the injured animal until you can get professional care. Our guidelines are based on what will happen with most dogs in most situations. However, there are always a few exceptions where the dog may not respond to your first aid as expected; these dogs will need professional care even sooner.

Contents

Published in Great Britain in 1982 by
Frederick Muller Ltd
Dataday House,
Wimbledon, London, SW19 7JU
in association with Charles Herridge Ltd
© Copyright 1981 by Publications International Ltd

Printed and bound in Great Britain
at The Pitman Press, Bath

ISBN 0 584 95016 0

About the Author: Sheldon Rubin, DVM is a practising veterinary surgeon in Chicago, USA. W. I. Atkinson, BVMS, MRCVS has a veterinary practice in North Devon.

Illustrations: Mike Muir
Cover Design: Frank E. Peiler

Contents

Dealing with an Emergency

Have you ever seen a dog injured in a fight or hit by a car? Perhaps you could only shake your head and walk away. Not because you didn't care, but because you didn't know how to approach and examine the dog, or what to do next. Especially if you have a dog of your own, you'll want to be prepared, for your dog depends on you for help in an emergency situation.

If we, like Dr. Doolittle, could "talk with the animals" it would be easy to find out what they had been doing, and where it hurt. Since we can't, in order to apply the proper treatment we must be able to identify signs that pinpoint the problem. The First Aid section of this book lists the most common emergencies alphabetically. When the nature of an injury or condition is not readily apparent, signs are listed at the beginning of the section to help you identify the problem.

The purpose of first aid is to relieve suffering and stabilize your dog's vital signs until professional help is obtained. This book will give you the information and techniques you'll need to confidently administer first aid, and perhaps save the life of a pet. Clear directions are listed step-by-step. Where more than one procedure is necessary to perform a step, each specific action is described in sub-steps "a, b, c, etc." An example of this occurs in Step 6 of SHOCK. These directions are further clarified with dozens of graphic illustrations.

The "why" of these procedures is explained in the back of the book. This section also includes preventive measures that can eliminate or minimize some hazards that could be dangerous to your pet.

The Index is cross-referenced to make it easy to find the page you need. Many emergency conditions will be found under several different headings. For example: "Freezing" will give you the page for "Hypothermia." "Snakebite" will also be listed under "Bites, poisonous snake," "Bites, nonpoisonous snake," "Poisonous snakebite," and "Nonpoisonous snakebite."

Because minutes count in an emergency situation, you'll want to have a first aid kit prepared. It needn't be elaborate; suggested items are listed on page 95. Keep the kit and this book together in a convenient place, and take both with you when you travel with your dog. Accidents often occur when you're far from home.

We suggest you take the time to thoroughly familiarize yourself with the contents of this book. Certain sections are especially important. When a dog is choking or unconscious, speed is vital if the dog is to live. Therefore, it is of primary importance that you know how to give artificial respiration and CPR (cardiopulmonary resuscitation). It will also be most helpful if you know exactly how to approach and restrain a dog if an accident does occur. Again, minutes count.

In addition to the information you will need to contact your veterinary surgeon, the police, or R.S.P.C.A. inspector. You will find the telephone numbers in your Yellow Pages telephone directory.

EMERGENCY INFORMATION

VETERINARY SURGEON'S NAME:_____

SURGERY PHONE:_____

EMERGENCY PHONE:_____

SURGERY ADDRESS:_____

R.S.P.C.A. PHONE:_____

Restraining an Injured Dog

STEP 1: **Approach slowly, speaking in a reassuring tone of voice.**

STEP 2: **Move close to the dog without touching it.**

STEP 3: **Stoop down to the dog. While continuing to speak, observe its eyes and facial expression.**

a. If the dog is wide-eyed and growling, DO NOT attempt to pet it. Proceed to Step 4.

b. If the dog is shivering, with its head lowered and a "smiling" appearance to its mouth, pet the dog for reassurance, first under the jaw. If this is permitted, pet the dog on the head.

STEP 4: **Slip a leash around the dog's neck. Use whatever material is available—rope, tie, belt, or torn rags.**

STEP 5: **If you are alone, place the leash around a fixed object, such as a fence post. Pull the dog against this object and tie the leash so the dog cannot move its head.**

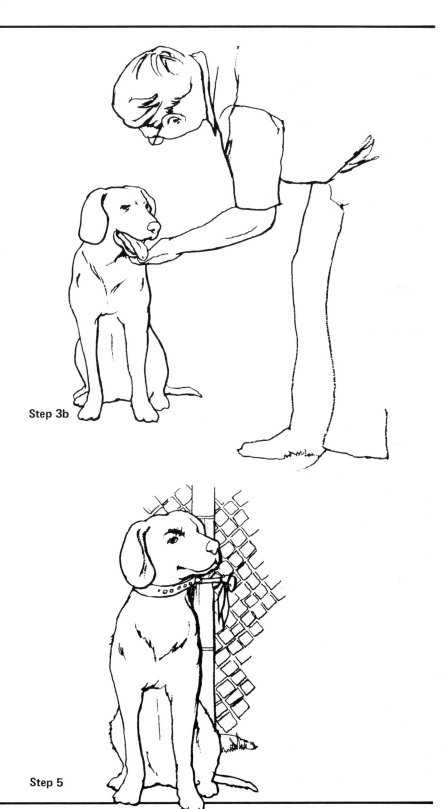

Step 3b

Step 5

STEP 6: Muzzle the dog to protect yourself. If the dog is very short-muzzled, proceed to Step 7.

a. Using a long piece of rope, torn rags, or a tie, loop over the dog's muzzle and tie a single knot under the chin.

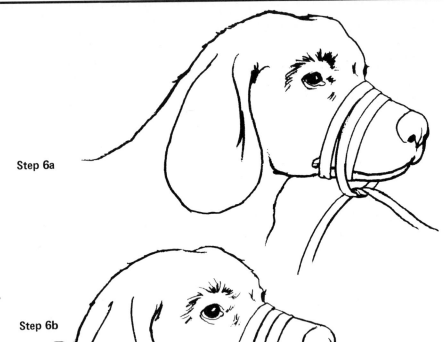

Step 6a

b. Bring the ends behind the ears and tie them in a bow.

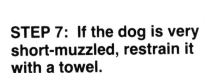

Step 6b

STEP 7: If the dog is very short-muzzled, restrain it with a towel.

a. Wrap the towel around the dog's neck and hold the towel in front of its head.

b. If you are alone, pin the towel in place.

STEP 8: If you are alone, proceed to administer treatment.

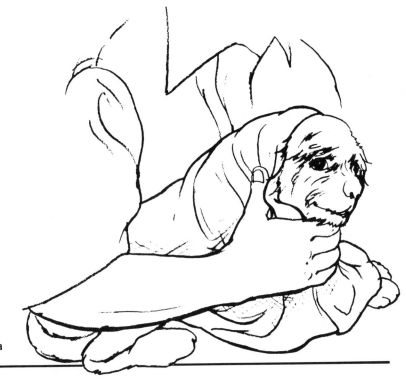

Step 7a

If you have an assistant

STEP 9: If possible, place the dog on a table or other raised surface.

a. If the dog is small, grasp its collar with one hand and place your other arm over its back and around its body. At the same time, pull forward on the collar and lift the dog's body, cradling it against your body.

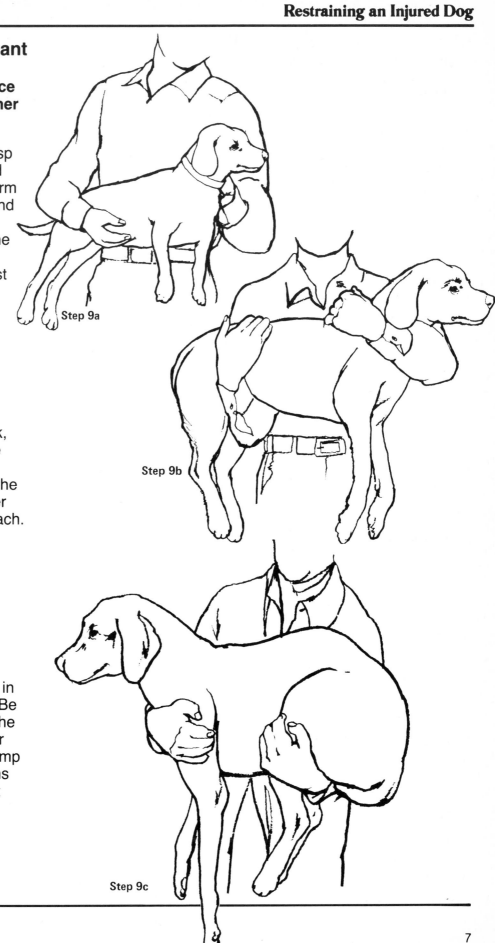

Step 9a

b. If the dog is large, slip one arm under its neck, holding its throat in the crook of your arm. Be sure the dog can breathe easily. Place your other arm under dog's stomach. Lift with both arms.

Step 9b

c. If the dog is very large, slip one arm under its neck, holding its throat in the crook of your arm. Be sure the dog can breathe easily. Place your other arm under the dog's rump and, pressing your arms toward one another, lift the dog.

Step 9c

STEP 10: If you want the dog on its side:

a. Stand or kneel so the dog is in front of you with its head to your right.

b. Reach over the dog's back and grasp the front leg closest to you with your right hand, and the rear leg closest to you with your left hand.

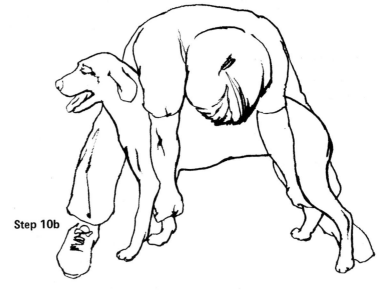

Step 10b

c. Push the dog's legs away from you and slide the dog down your body.

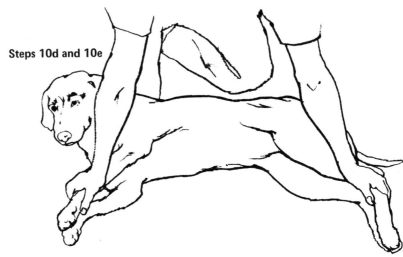

Steps 10d and 10e

d. Grasp both front legs in your right hand and both rear legs in your left hand.

e. Hold the dog's neck down gently with your right arm.

f. Have your assistant administer treatment.

STEP 11: If you want the dog sitting:

a. Slip one arm under the dog's neck, holding its throat in the crook of your arm. Be sure the dog can breathe easily.

b. Place your other arm over the dog's back and around its stomach.

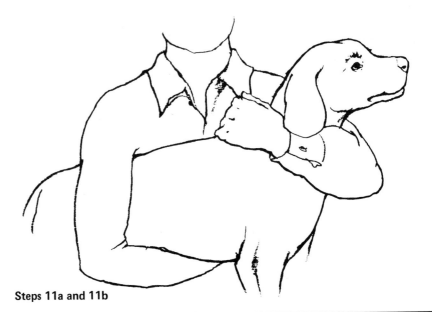

Steps 11a and 11b

c. Pressing the dog against your body, apply body weight to the dog's rear quarters.

d. Have your assistant administer treatment.

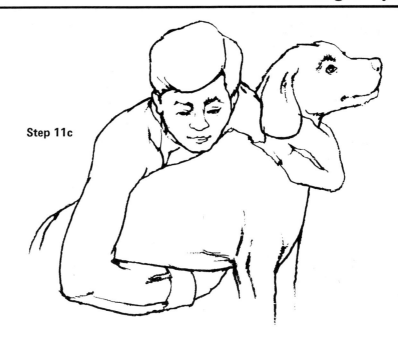

Step 11c

STEP 12: If you want the dog standing:

a. Slip one arm under the dog's neck, holding its throat in the crook of your arm. Be sure the dog can breathe easily.

b. Place your other arm under the dog's stomach.

c. Press the dog toward your body and lift upward.

d. Have your assistant administer treatment.

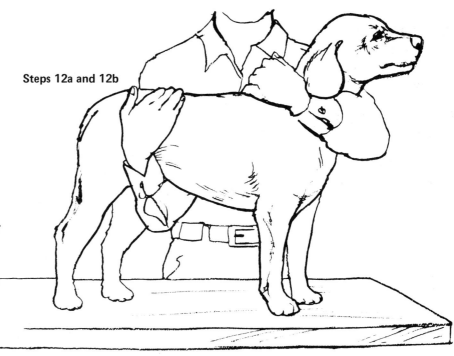

Steps 12a and 12b

Transporting an Injured Dog

A. If the dog can be lifted

STEP 1: If the dog is small:

a. Grasp its collar with one hand and place your other arm over its back and around its body.

b. At the same time, pull forward on the collar and lift the dog's body, cradling it against your body.

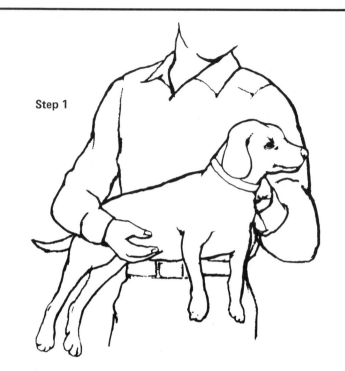

Step 1

STEP 2: If the dog is large:

a. Slip one arm under its neck, holding its throat in the crook of your arm. Be sure the dog can breathe easily.

b. Place your other arm under the dog's stomach. Lift with both arms.

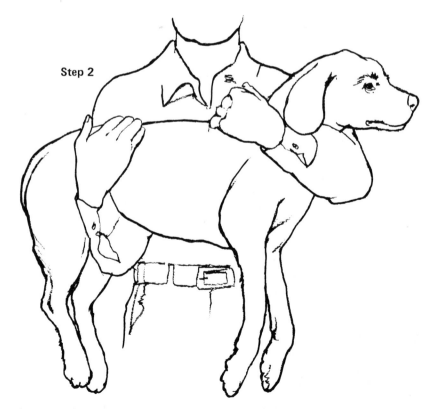

Step 2

STEP 3: If the dog is very large:

a. Slip one arm under its neck, holding its throat in the crook of your arm. Be sure the dog can breathe easily.

b. Place your other arm under the dog's rump and, pressing your arms toward one another, lift the dog.

STEP 4: Telephone your veterinary surgeon and take the dog to the surgery.

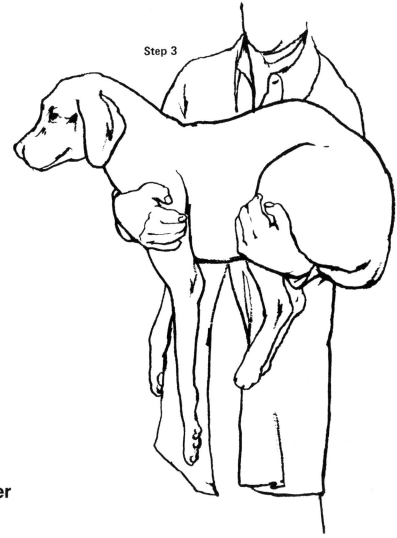

Step 3

B. If the dog needs a stretcher

> A flat board must be used if a broken back is suspected.

STEP 1: Use a blanket or flat board as a stretcher. If you are using a board proceed to Step 2. If you are using a blanket:

a. Place one hand under the dog's chest and the other under its rear; carefully lift or slide the dog onto the blanket.

b. Telephone your veterinary surgeon and take the dog to the surgery.

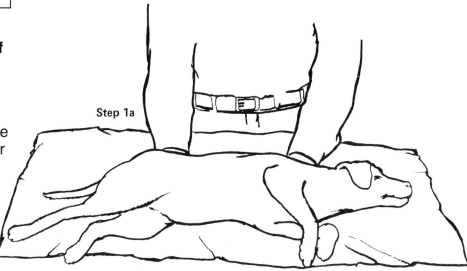

Step 1a

STEP 2: If you are using a flat board:

a. Depending on the size of the dog, use a table leaf, ironing board, TV table top, large cutting board, or removable bookshelf. Make sure whatever you use will fit in your car.

b. Place two or three long strips of cloth or rope equidistant under the board, avoiding the area where the dog's neck will rest.

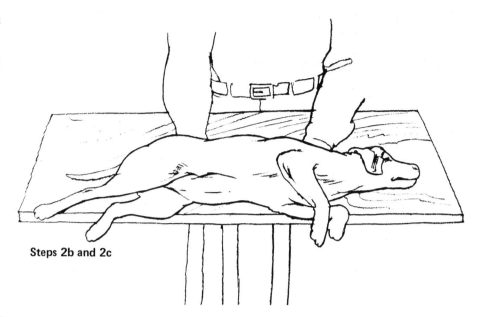

Steps 2b and 2c

c. Place one hand under the dog's chest and the other under its rear; carefully lift or slide the dog onto the board.

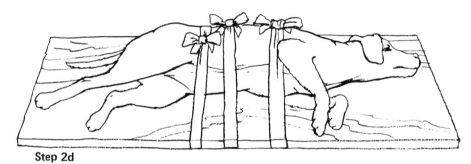

Step 2d

d. Tie the dog to the board.

e. Telephone your veterinary surgeon and take the dog to the surgery.

Administering Oral Medicine

A. Liquids

STEP 1: If you have an assistant, restrain the dog.

a. Relieve the dog's apprehension by talking quietly and reassuringly.

b. Slip one arm under the dog's neck, holding its throat gently in the crook of your arm. Be sure the dog can breathe easily.

c. Pass the other arm over or under the middle of the dog, using gentle but firm pressure to hold its body against yours.

d. If necessary, apply a mouth-tie loosely so there is only slight jaw movement. See page 6.

STEP 2: Gently tip the dog's head slightly backwards.

STEP 3: Pull the lower lip out at the corner to make a pouch.

STEP 4: Using a measuring spoon or dose syringe, place the fluid a little at a time into the pouch, allowing each small amount to be swallowed before giving any more of the dose.

> If the dog is hard to handle, you will need help restraining it.

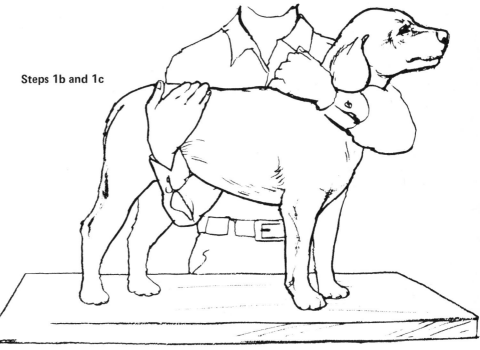

Steps 1b and 1c

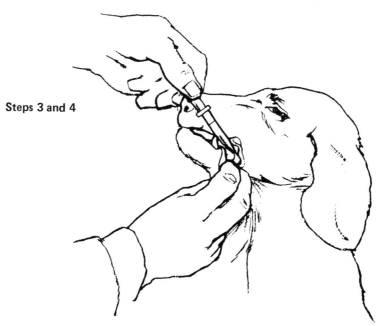

Steps 3 and 4

STEP 5: Gently rub the throat to stimulate swallowing.

Step 5

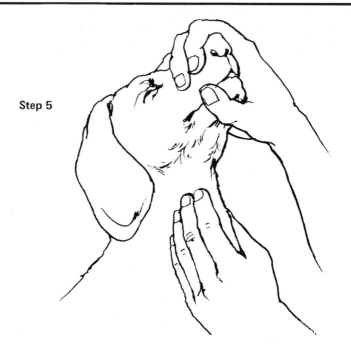

B. Pills

STEP 1: If you have an assistant, restrain the dog.

a. Relieve the dog's apprehension by talking quietly and reassuringly.

b. Slip one arm under the dog's neck, holding its throat gently in the crook of your arm. Be sure the dog can breathe easily.

c. Pass the other arm over or under the middle of the dog, using gentle but firm pressure to hold its body against yours.

Steps 1b and 1c

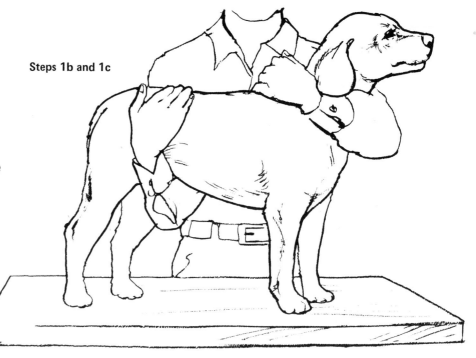

STEP 2: Grasp the dog's upper jaw with one hand over its muzzle.

STEP 3: Press the lips over the upper teeth by pressing your thumb on one side and your fingers on the other so the dog's lips are between its teeth and your fingers. Firm pressure will force the mouth open.

STEP 4: Hold the pill between the thumb and index finger of your other hand and place the pill as far back in the mouth as possible.

STEP 5: Gently rub the dog's throat to stimulate swallowing.

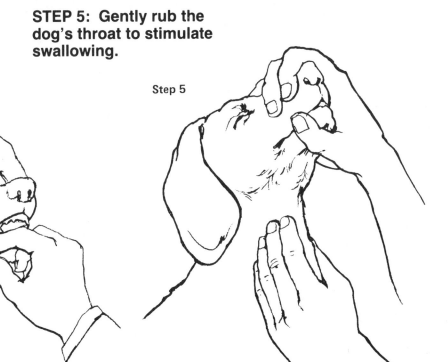

Steps 2, 3, and 4

Step 5

Animal Bite

STEP 1: Restrain the dog if necessary. See page 5.

STEP 2: Clip the hair around the wound.

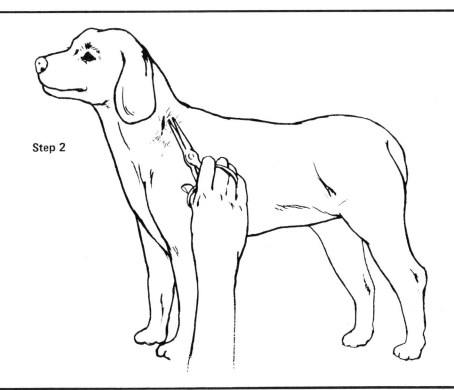

Step 2

STEP 3: Flush thoroughly by pouring 3% (10 volumes) hydrogen peroxide or weak salt solution (1 teaspoon of salt to 1 pint of water) into the wound. DO NOT use any other antiseptic.

STEP 4: Examine the wound. If the tissue under the wound appears to pass by when you move the skin, the wound will probably require stitches.

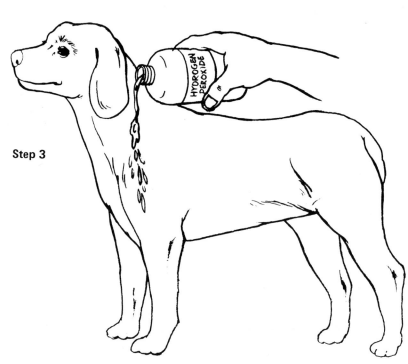

Step 3

STEP 5: DO NOT bandage. Allow the wound to drain unless there is excessive bleeding. If the wound does bleed excessively, follow these steps:

a. Cover wound with clean cloth or sterile dressing.

b. Place your hand over the dressing and press firmly.

c. Keep pressure on the dressing to stop bleeding.

d. If blood soaks through the dressing, DO NOT remove. Apply more dressing and continue to apply pressure until bleeding stops.

STEP 6: If the wound is deep enough to require stitches, transport immediately to the veterinary surgeon.

Step 5: Stop bleeding only if the wound bleeds excessively.

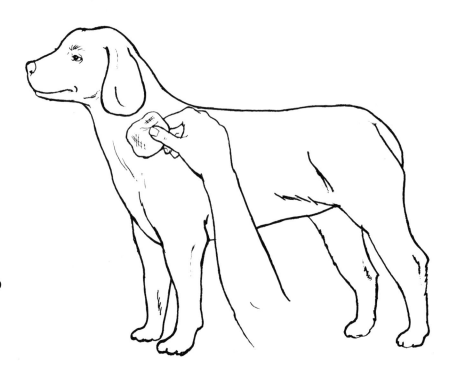

Spurting Blood

WATCH FOR SIGNS OF SHOCK:

Pale or white gums, rapid heartbeat and breathing. If signs are present see page 71.

If any wound is spurting blood, it means an artery has been cut. This requires immediate professional attention.

A. On head or torso

STEP 1: Restrain the dog if necessary. See page 5.

STEP 2: Cover the wound with a clean folded towel or sterile dressing.

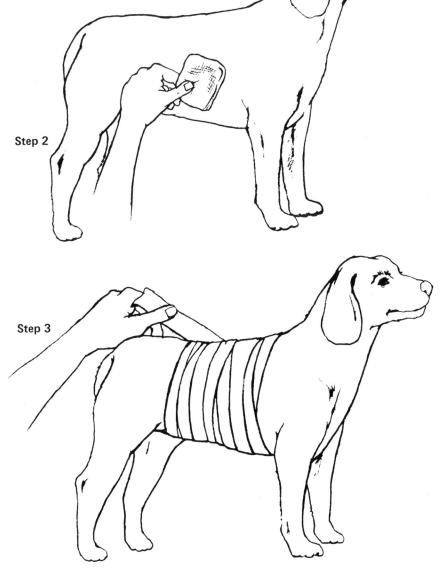

Step 2

STEP 3: Wrap torn rags or other soft material around the dressing and tie or tape just tightly enough to hold in place.

STEP 4: Telephone your veterinary surgeon and take the dog to the surgery.

Step 3

B. On legs or tail

STEP 1: Restrain the dog if necessary. See page 5.

STEP 2: Apply a tourniquet.

a. Use a tie, belt, or piece of cloth folded to about one inch width. DO NOT use rope, wire, or string.

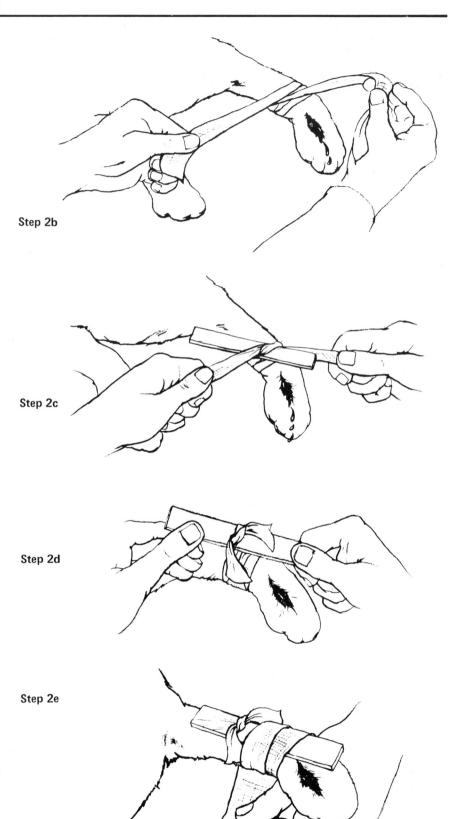

Step 2b

b. Place the material between the wound and the heart, an inch or two above, but not touching, the wound.

Step 2c

c. Tie a stick or ruler to the material with a single knot.

d. Twist the stick until bleeding stops, but no tighter.

Step 2d

e. Wrap a piece of cloth around the stick and limb to keep in place.

Step 2e

STEP 3: If it will take time to reach the veterinary surgeon, loosen the tourniquet every 15 minutes for a period of 1-2 minutes and then tighten again.

STEP 4: Telephone your veterinary surgeon and take the dog to the surgery.

Internal Bleeding

SIGNS: PALE OR WHITE GUMS; RAPID HEARTBEAT AND BREATHING; AVAILABILITY OF RAT OR MOUSE POISON; BLEEDING FROM THE EARS, NOSE, OR MOUTH WITH ANY OF THE ABOVE SIGNS.

STEP 1: If there is bleeding from any external wounds, treat for shock. See page 71.

STEP 2: Place the dog on its side with its head extended.

STEP 3: Gently pull out the dog's tongue to keep the airway open.

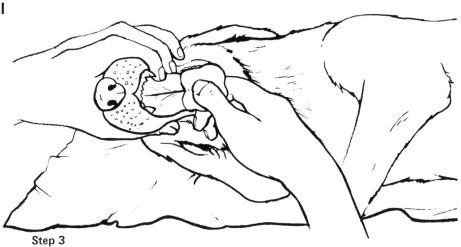

Step 3

STEP 4: Elevate the dog's hindquarters slightly by placing them on a pillow or folded towels.

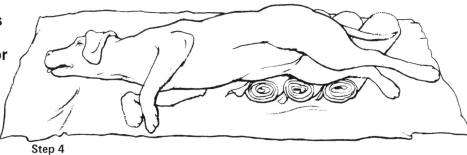

Step 4

STEP 5: To conserve body heat, place a hot water bottle (100°F/37°C) against the abdomen. Wrap the bottle in cloth to prevent burns.

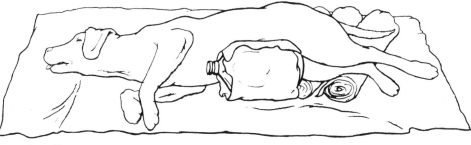

Step 5

Step 6

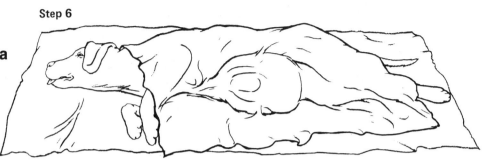

STEP 6: Wrap the dog in a blanket or jacket.

STEP 7: Telephone your veterinary surgeon and take the dog to the surgery.

Bleeding Chest or Abdomen

WATCH FOR SIGNS OF SHOCK: Pale or white gums, rapid heartbeat and breathing. If signs are present see page 71.

STEP 1: Restrain the dog if necessary. See page 5.

STEP 2: If the wound is in the chest and a "sucking" noise is heard, bandage tightly enough to keep air from entering and transport immediately to the veterinary surgeon.

STEP 3: If there is a protruding object, such as an arrow, see page 67.

Step 3

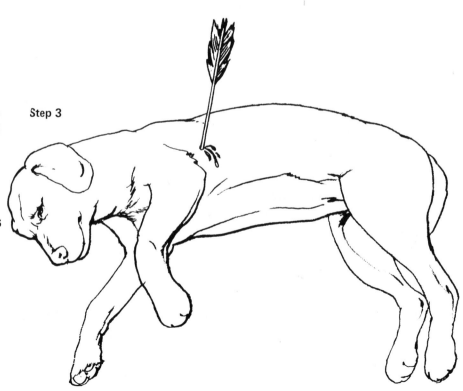

STEP 4: Clip the hair around the injured area.

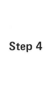

Step 4

STEP 5: Examine the wound for glass or other foreign objects. If visible, remove with fingers or tweezers. If the tissue under the wound appears to pass by when you move the skin, the wound will probably require stitches.

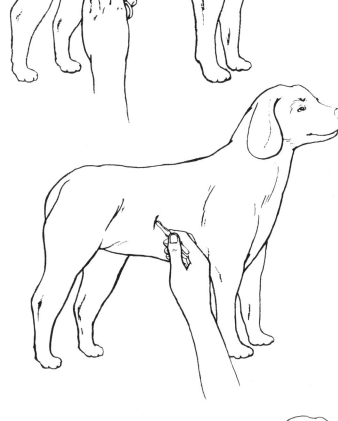

Step 5

STEP 6: Flush thoroughly by pouring 3% (10 volumes) hydrogen peroxide or weak salt solution (1 teaspoon of salt to 1 pint of water) into wound. DO NOT use any other antiseptic.

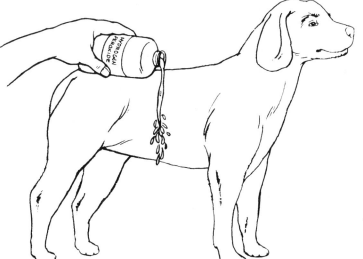

Step 6

STEP 7: Cover the wound with a clean cloth or sterile dressing.

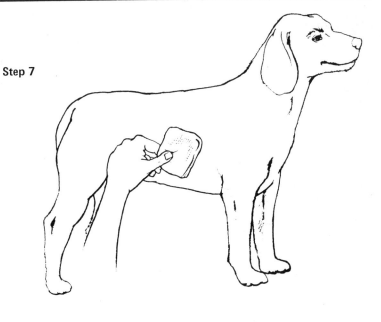

Step 7

STEP 8: Place your hand over the dressing and press firmly.

STEP 9: Keep pressure on the dressing to stop bleeding. If blood soaks through the dressing, DO NOT remove. Apply more dressing and continue to apply pressure until bleeding stops.

Step 10

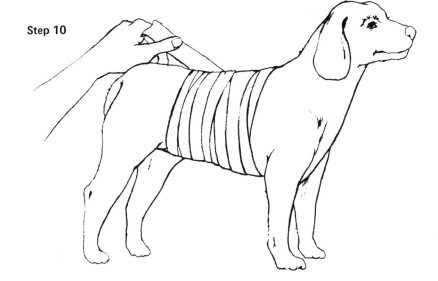

STEP 10: Wrap torn sheets or other soft material around the dressing and tie or tape just tightly enough to keep the bandage on.

STEP 11: If the wound is deep enough to require stitches, telephone your veterinary surgeon and take the dog to the surgery.

Bleeding
Ear

Cut ears bleed profusely.

STEP 1: Restrain the dog if necessary. See page 5.

STEP 2: Cover the wound with a clean cloth or sterile dressing. Place dressing material on both sides of the ear flap, then fold over the top of the dog's head and hold firmly to control bleeding.

Step 2

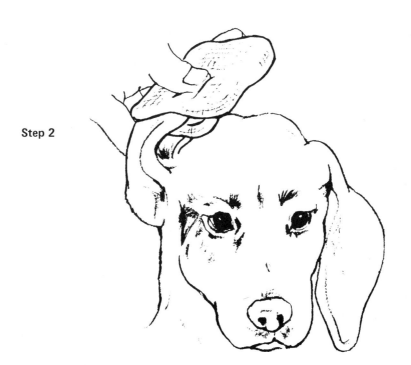

Step 3

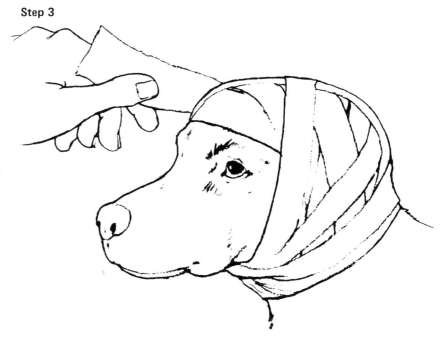

STEP 3: Wrap torn sheets or rags around the dressing, ear, and head, making sure the entire ear is covered. Tape or tie in place.

STEP 4: Telephone your veterinary surgeon and take the dog to the surgery.

Bleeding Leg, Paw, or Tail

WATCH FOR SIGNS OF SHOCK: Pale or white gums, rapid heartbeat and breathing. If signs are present see page 71.

STEP 1: Restrain the dog if necessary. See page 5.

STEP 2: Clip the hair around the injured area.

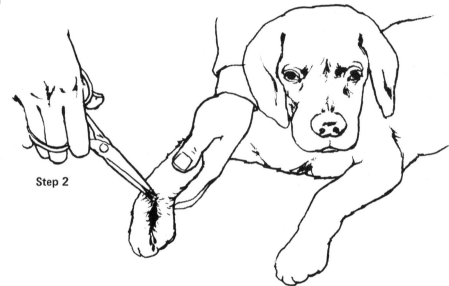

Step 2

STEP 3: Examine the wound for glass or other foreign objects. If visible, remove with fingers or tweezers. If the tissue under the wound appears to pass by when you move the skin, the wound will probably require stitches.

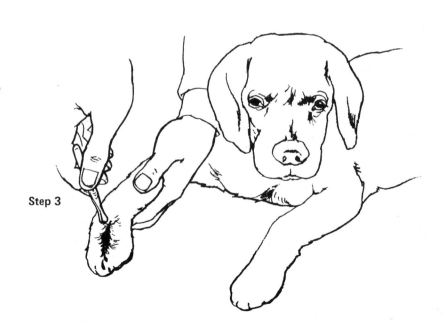

Step 3

STEP 4: Flush thoroughly by pouring 3% (10 volumes) hydrogen peroxide or weak salt solution (1 teaspoon of salt to 1 pint of water) into the wound. DO NOT use any other antiseptic.

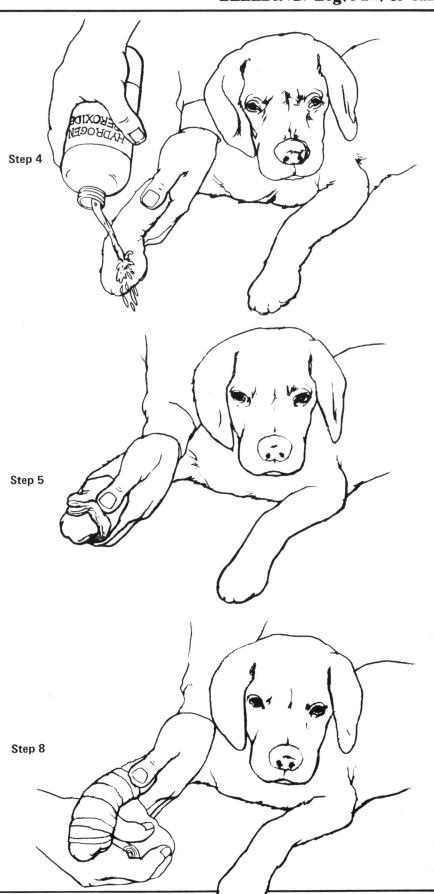

Step 4

STEP 5: Cover the wound with a clean cloth or sterile dressing.

STEP 6: Place your hand over the dressing and press firmly.

STEP 7: Keep pressure on the dressing to stop bleeding. If blood soaks through the dressing, DO NOT remove. Apply more dressing and continue to apply pressure until bleeding stops. If bleeding does not stop within 5 minutes, proceed to Step 10.

Step 5

STEP 8: Wrap torn rags or other soft material around the dressing and tie or tape just tightly enough to keep the bandage on. Start below the wound and wrap upward.

Step 8

STEP 9: If the wound is deep enough to require stitches, keep the dog off the injured leg and after telephoning your veterinary surgeon take the dog to the surgery.

STEP 10: If bleeding does not stop within 5 minutes, apply a tourniquet.

a. Use a tie, belt, or piece of cloth folded to about one inch width. DO NOT use rope, wire, or string.

b. Place the material between the wound and the heart, an inch or two above, but not touching, the wound.

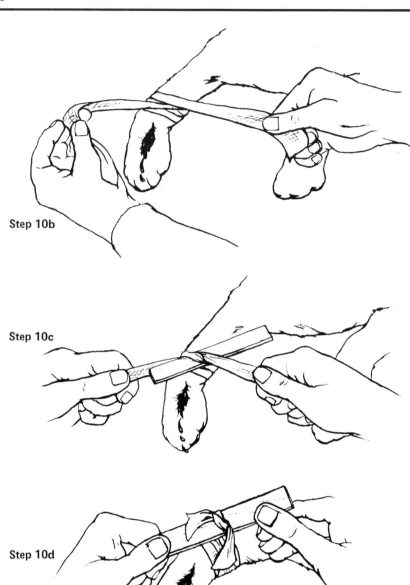

Step 10b

Step 10c

c. Tie a stick or ruler to the material with a single knot.

d. Twist the stick until bleeding stops, but no tighter.

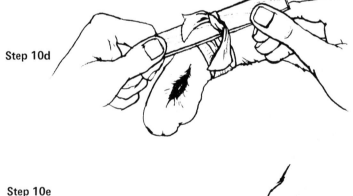

Step 10d

e. Wrap a piece of cloth around the stick and limb to keep in place.

Step 10e

STEP 11: If it will take time to reach the veterinary surgeon, loosen the tourniquet every 15 minutes for a period of 1-2 minutes and then tighten again.

STEP 12: Telephone your veterinary surgeon and take the dog to the surgery immediately.

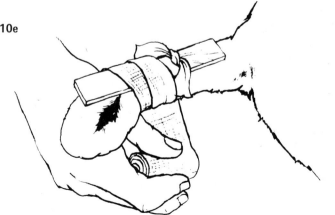

Bleeding
Nail

A. Nail broken

STEP 1: Restrain the dog if necessary. See page 5.

STEP 2: DO NOT try to cut or remove the broken nail.

STEP 3: Hold a clean cloth or sterile dressing against the nail. Bleeding will stop in a few minutes.

STEP 4: Telephone your veterinary surgeon and take the dog to the surgery.

Step 3

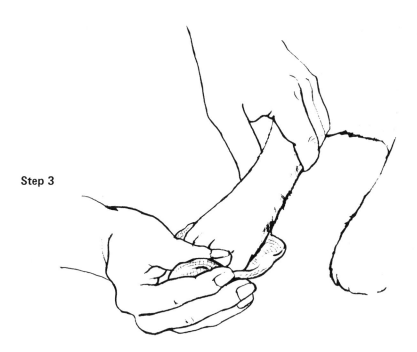

B. Nail cut too short

STEP 1: Restrain the dog if necessary. See page 5.

STEP 2: Hold a clean cloth or sterile dressing against the nail.

STEP 3: Keep firm pressure on the area for at least 5 minutes. DO NOT remove until bleeding stops.

STEP 4: If bleeding does not stop in 15-20 minutes, telephone your veterinary surgeon as soon as possible. Continuous bleeding indicates a bleeding disorder that should be treated promptly.

Step 2

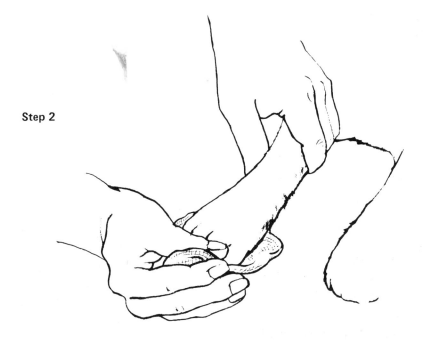

Bleeding Nose

STEP 1: Restrain the dog if necessary, but DO NOT tie its mouth shut. See page 5.

STEP 2: Apply ice packs to the top of the dog's nose between its eyes and nostrils.

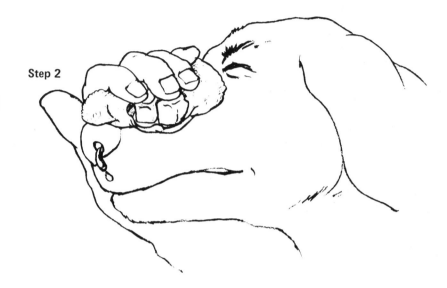

Step 2

STEP 3: Cover the bleeding nostril with a clean cloth or sterile dressing.

STEP 4: Hold firmly until bleeding stops.

STEP 5: If the nostril was not cut, a bloody nose in a dog could indicate a serious disorder. Contact your veterinary surgeon immediately.

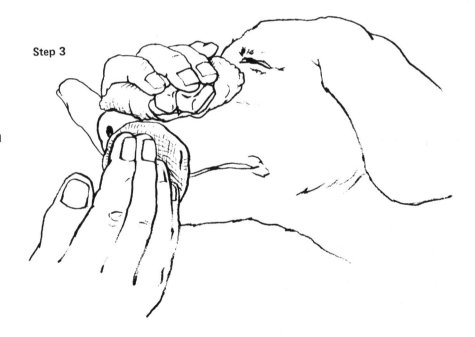

Step 3

Bloat

SIGNS: EXCESSIVE DROOLING, PACING AND AGITATION, ENLARGED ABDOMEN, FREQUENT ATTEMPTS TO VOMIT PRODUCING LARGE AMOUNTS OF WHITE FOAM OR NOTHING AT ALL. USUALLY SEEN IN LARGE, DEEP-CHESTED DOGS.

STEP 1: Telephone and take your dog immediately to your veterinary surgeon. Bloat is frequently followed by gastric torsion (turning of the stomach), which leads to shock and death in a matter of a few hours. **DO NOT DELAY** in contacting your veterinary surgeon as the condition of your dog can deteriorate very quickly.

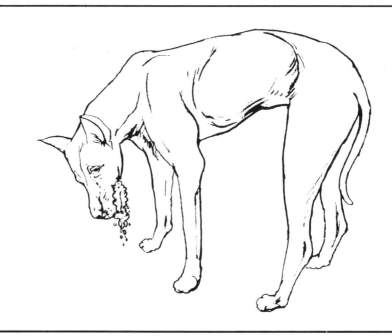

Broken Back

SIGNS: PARALYSIS, UNUSUAL ARCH TO BACK, EXTREME PAIN IN BACK AREA.

WATCH FOR SIGNS OF SHOCK: Pale or white gums, rapid heartbeat and breathing. If signs are present see page 71.

STEP 1: Muzzle the dog if necessary. See page 6.

STEP 2: If you suspect a broken back, lift the dog onto a flat board without bending its back. **DO NOT** attempt to splint.

a. Depending on the size of the dog, use a table leaf, ironing board, TV table top, large cutting board, or removable bookshelf. Make sure whatever you use will fit in your car.

b. Place two or three long strips of cloth or rope equidistant under the board.

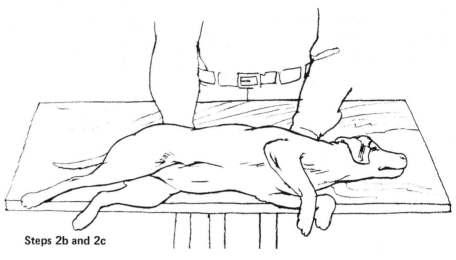

Steps 2b and 2c

c. Place one hand under the dog's chest and the other under its rear section and carefully lift or slide it onto the board.

d. Tie the dog onto the board.

STEP 3: Telephone your veterinary surgeon and take the dog to the surgery.

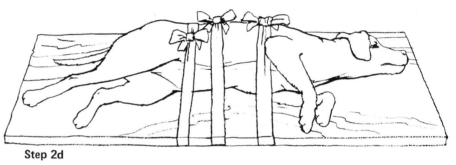

Step 2d

Broken Leg

SIGNS: LEG IS MISSHAPEN, HANGS LIMPLY, CANNOT SUPPORT BODY WEIGHT; SUDDEN ONSET OF PAIN IN AREA; SWELLING.

WATCH FOR SIGNS OF SHOCK:

Pale or white gums, rapid heartbeat and breathing. If signs are present see page 71.

STEP 1: Restrain the dog if necessary. See page 5.

STEP 2: Examine the leg and determine if the fracture is open (wound near the break or bone protruding from the skin) or closed (no break in the skin).

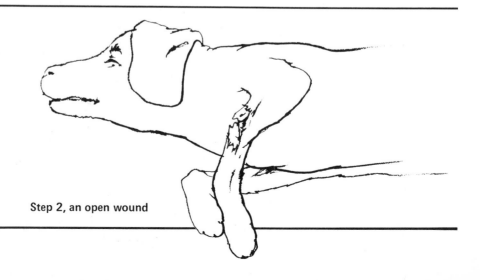

Step 2, an open wound

STEP 3: If the fracture is closed, proceed to Step 4. If the fracture is open:

a. Flush thoroughly by pouring 3% (10 volumes) hydrogen peroxide into the wound. If this is not available DO NOT use any other antiseptic but proceed to b.

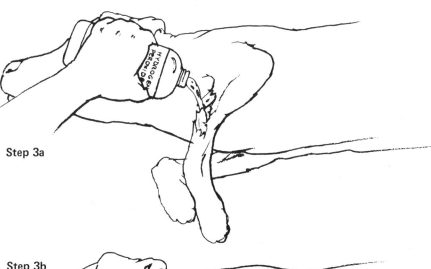

Step 3a

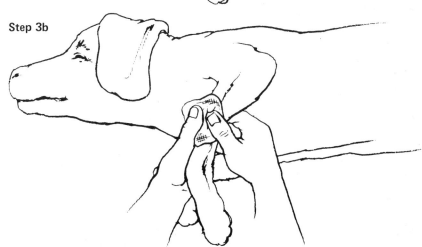

Step 3b

b. Cover the wound with a sterile bandage or clean cloth.

c. DO NOT attempt to splint the fracture. Hold a large folded towel under the unsplinted limb and after telephoning the veterinary surgeon, take the dog to the surgery immediately.

Step 3c

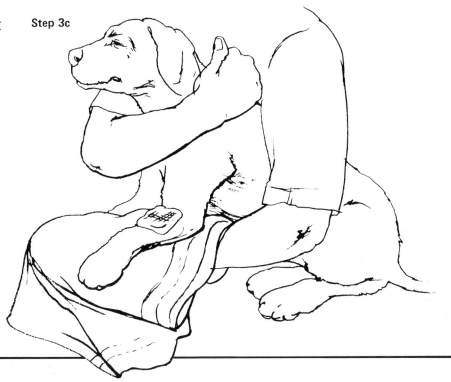

STEP 4: If the broken limb is grossly misshapen or the dog appears to be in great pain when you attempt to splint, stop and proceed to Step 5. Otherwise, proceed to splint the bone.

a. Use any splint material available—sticks, newspaper, magazine, or stiff cardboard. The object is to immobilize the limb, not reset it.

Step 4a

Step 4a

b. Attach the splints to the fractured leg with torn strips of cloth or gauze.

c. Tape or tie firmly, but not so tightly that circulation may be impaired.

d. Contact your veterinary surgeon and take the dog to the surgery.

Step 4c

STEP 5: If the broken limb is grossly misshapen or the dog appears to be in great pain when you attempt to splint, hold a large towel under the unsplinted limb for support and, after telephoning the veterinary surgeon, take the dog to the surgery immediately.

Step 5

Broken Ribs

SIGNS: UNUSUAL SHAPE OF RIB CAGE, EXTREME PAIN IN CHEST AREA.

WATCH FOR SIGNS OF SHOCK: Pale or white gums, rapid heartbeat and breathing. If signs are present see page 71.

A. If broken ribs are obvious or suspected

STEP 1: Restrain the dog if necessary. See page 5.

STEP 2: Wrap torn sheets or gauze around the entire chest area to immobilize.

STEP 3: Telephone the veterinary surgeon and take the dog to the surgery.

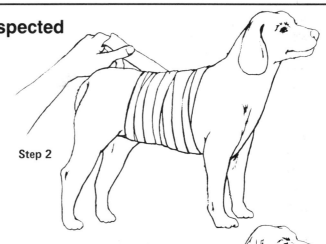

Step 2

B. If the side of the chest bulges as the dog breathes

A bulging chest usually means there is deep muscle damage to the chest wall that requires immediate professional attention.

STEP 1: Restrain the dog if necessary. See page 5.

STEP 2: Place a thick folded cloth over the bulge.

STEP 3: Bandage with torn cloth or gauze, tightly enough to keep pressure on the bulge.

STEP 4: Telephone the veterinary surgeon and take the dog to the surgery immediately.

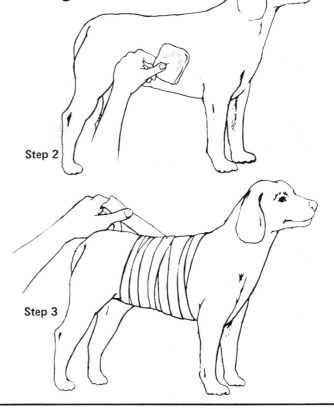

Step 2

Step 3

First or Second Degree Burns

**SIGNS: 1ST DEGREE—FUR INTACT OR SINGED, PAINFUL LESION, SKIN RED WITH POSSIBLE BLISTERS.
2ND DEGREE—SINGED FUR, PAINFUL LESION WHICH TURNS DRY AND TAN IN COLOUR, SWELLING.**

STEP 1: Restrain the dog if necessary. See page 5.

STEP 2: Apply cold water or ice packs to the burned area and leave in contact with the skin for 15 minutes. DO NOT apply ointment or butter.

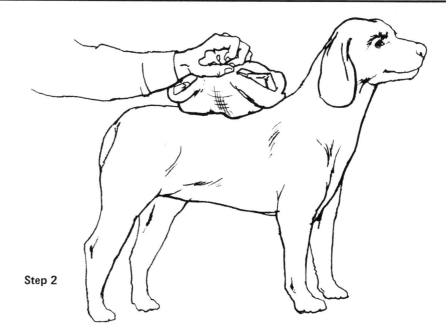

Step 2

STEP 3: If burns cover a large part of the body or are located where the dog can lick them, cover with a sterile dressing. DO NOT use cotton.

STEP 4: Telephone the veterinary surgeon and take the dog to the surgery as soon as possible.

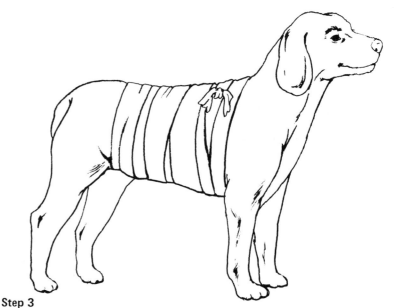

Step 3

Third Degree Burns

SIGNS: PROBABLE SHOCK IF EXTENSIVE BODY AREA IS INVOLVED, DESTRUCTION OF ENTIRE SKIN AREA, BLACK OR PURE WHITE LESION, FUR PULLS OUT EASILY.

STEP 1: Restrain the dog if necessary. See page 5.

STEP 2: Examine for shock. See page 71.

STEP 3: Apply a dry, clean dressing over the burned area. DO NOT use cotton.

STEP 4: Telephone the veterinary surgeon and take the dog to the surgery immediately.

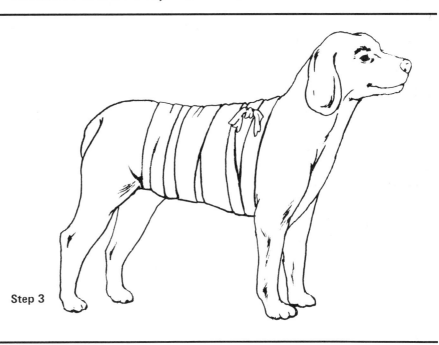

Step 3

Chemical Burns

SIGNS: CHEMICAL ODOUR SUCH AS TURPENTINE, PETROL, OR INSECTICIDE; REDDENED SKIN; PAIN.

STEP 1: Restrain the dog if necessary. See page 5.

STEP 2: Wash the area thoroughly with soap and water; repeat as many times as necessary to remove the chemical. Use mild soap and lather well. DO NOT use solvents of any kind.

STEP 3: Call the veterinary surgeon for further instructions.

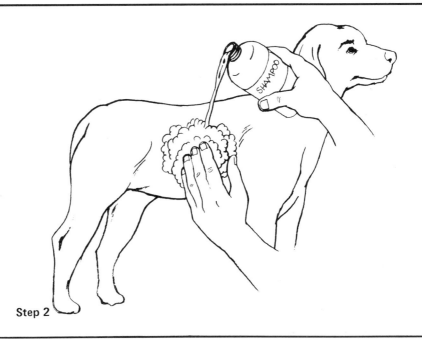

Step 2

Choking

SIGNS: PAWING AT MOUTH, PALE OR BLUE TONGUE, OBVIOUS DISTRESS, UNCONSCIOUSNESS.

STEP 1: Restrain the dog if necessary; DO NOT tie its mouth shut. See page 5.

STEP 2: Clear the airway.

a. Open the mouth carefully by grasping the upper jaw with one hand over the muzzle.

b. Press the lips over the upper teeth by pressing your thumb on one side and your fingers on the other so that the lips are between the dog's teeth and your fingers. Firm pressure will force the mouth open.

c. If you can see the object, try to remove it with your fingers.

d. If you cannot remove the object and the dog is small enough, pick it up by grasping its back legs; turn it upside down and shake vigorously. Slapping the back while shaking may help to dislodge the object.

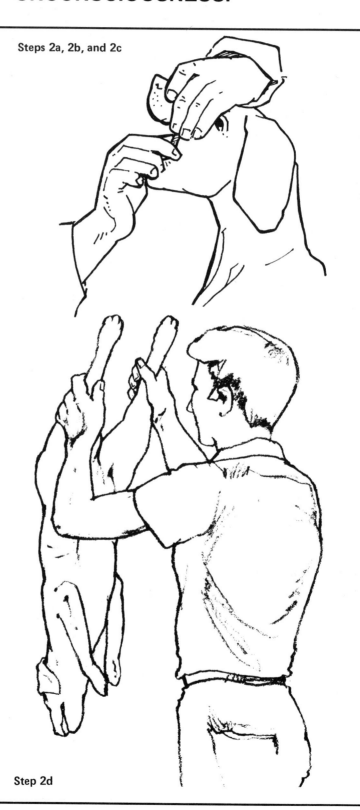

Steps 2a, 2b, and 2c

Step 2d

e. If you cannot remove the object and the dog is too large to pick up, place the dog on its side on the floor. Place your hand just behind the rib cage and press down and slightly forward quickly and firmly. Release. Repeat rapidly several times until the object is expelled.

STEP 3: If you cannot dislodge the object, contact your veterinary surgeon and take the dog to the surgery immediately.

STEP 4: If you dislodge the object and the dog is not breathing, feel for heartbeat by placing fingers about 2 inches behind the dog's elbow in the middle of its chest.

STEP 5: If the heart is not beating, proceed to Step 6. If it is, perform artificial respiration.

a. Turn the dog on its side.

b. Hold the dog's mouth and lips closed and blow firmly into its nostrils. Blow for 3 seconds, take a deep breath, and repeat until you feel resistance or see the chest rise.

c. After 1 minute, stop. Watch the chest for movement to indicate the dog is breathing on its own.

d. If the dog is not breathing, continue artificial respiration.

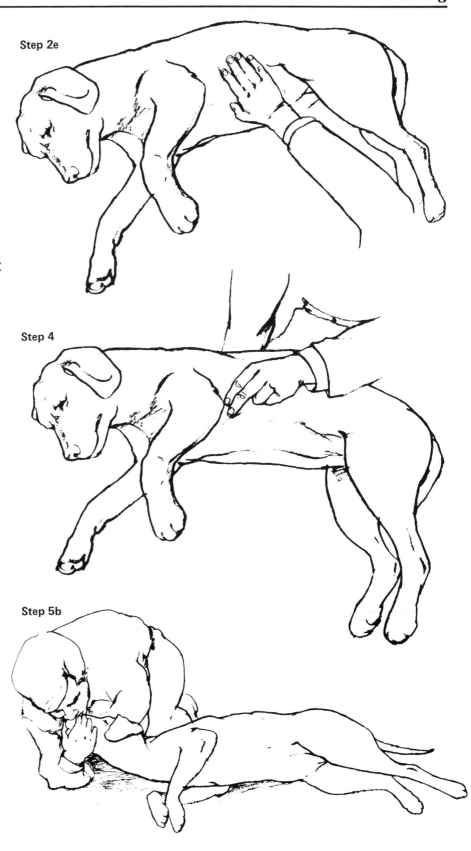

Step 2e

Step 4

Step 5b

STEP 6: If the heart is not beating, perform CPR (cardiopulmonary resuscitation).

CPR for dogs weighing up to 45 pounds

a. Turn the dog on its back.

b. Kneel down at the head of the dog.

c. Clasp your hands over the dog's chest with your palms resting on either side of its chest.

d. Compress your palms on the chest firmly for a count of "2" and release for a count of "1." Moderate pressure is required. Repeat about 30 times in 30 seconds.

e. Alternately (after 30 seconds), hold the dog's mouth and lips closed and blow firmly into its nostrils. Blow for 3 seconds, take a deep breath, and repeat until you feel resistance or see the chest rise. Try to repeat this 20 times in 60 seconds.

f. After 1 minute, stop. Look at the chest for breathing movement and feel for heartbeat by placing fingers about 2 inches behind the dog's elbow in the centre of its chest.

g. If the dog's heart is not beating, continue CPR. If the heart starts beating, but the dog is still not breathing, return to Step 5.

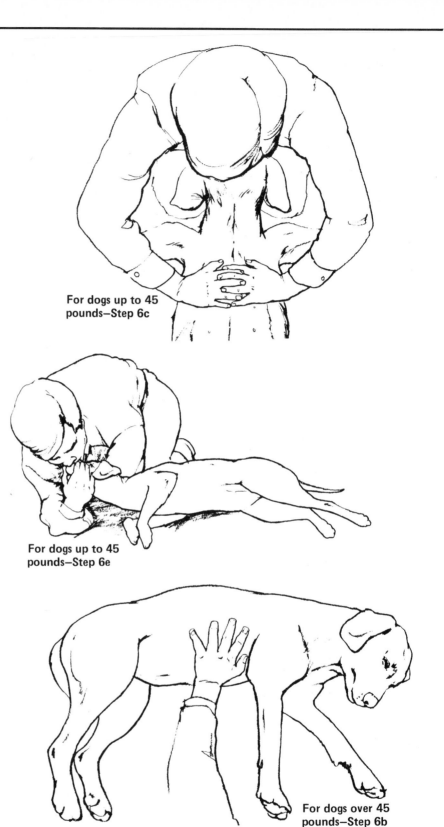

For dogs up to 45 pounds—Step 6c

For dogs up to 45 pounds—Step 6e

For dogs over 45 pounds—Step 6b

CPR for dogs weighing over 45 pounds

a. Turn the dog on its side.

b. Place the palm of your hand in the middle of the dog's chest.

c. Press for a count of "2" and release for a count of "1." Firm pressure is required. Repeat about 30 times in 30 seconds.

d. Alternately (after 30 seconds), hold the dog's mouth and lips closed and blow firmly into its nostrils. Blow for 3 seconds, take a deep breath, and repeat until you feel resistance or see the chest rise. Try to repeat this 20 times in 60 seconds.

e. After 1 minute, stop. Look at the chest for breathing movement and feel for heartbeat by placing fingers about 2 inches

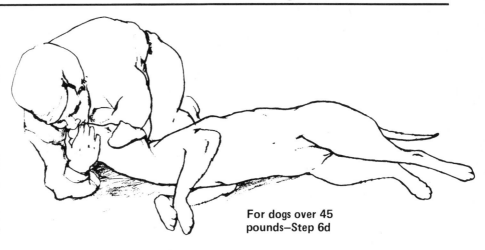

For dogs over 45 pounds—Step 6d

behind the dog's elbow in the centre of its chest.

f. If the dog's heart is not beating, continue CPR. If the heart starts beating, but the dog is still not breathing, return to Step 5.

STEP 7: Telephone the veterinary surgeon and take the dog to the surgery. CPR or artificial respiration should be continued on the way to the surgery or until dog is breathing and its heart is beating without assistance.

Convulsion/ Seizure

Be patient; do not panic. Convulsions are rarely fatal and most last only a few minutes.

STEP 1: DO NOT place your fingers or any object in the dog's mouth.

STEP 2: Pull the dog away from walls and furniture to prevent self-injury.

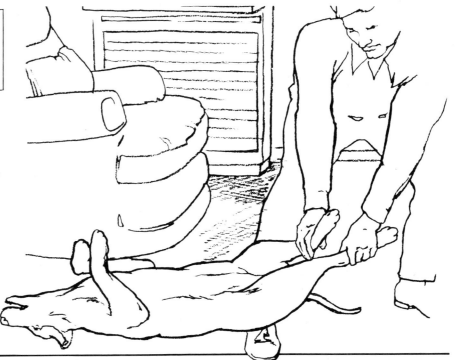

Step 2

STEP 3: Wrap the dog in a blanket to help protect it from injury.

STEP 4: When the seizure has stopped, contact the veterinary surgeon for further instructions.

STEP 5: If the seizure does not stop within 10 minutes, or if the dog comes out of the seizure and goes into another one within an hour, contact the veterinary surgeon immediately.

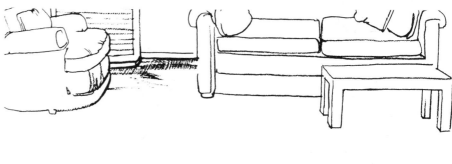
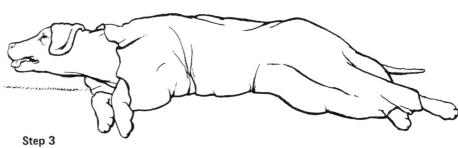
Step 3

Diarrhoea

STEP 1: Remove all food immediately. Water is important to prevent dehydration in severe diarrhoea. It should not be removed.

STEP 2: If blood appears or if diarrhoea continues for more than 24 hours, contact the veterinary surgeon. He will probably want to see a stool sample.

STEP 3: Treat with a kaolin pectin mixture every 4-6 hours at the rate of one teaspoon per 10-15 pounds of the dog's weight. See ADMINISTERING ORAL MEDICINE, page 13.

STEP 4: DO NOT attempt to feed for at least 12 hours.

STEP 5: After 12 hours, feed the dog a mixture of small quantities of boiled minced beef or mutton, cooked rice, and cottage cheese. This diet should be continued until stools are formed.

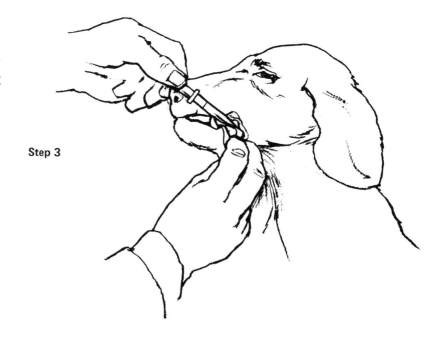
Step 3

Drowning

**WATCH FOR
SIGNS OF SHOCK:**
Pale or white gums, rapid heartbeat and breathing. If signs are present see page 71.

STEP 1: Rescue the dog.

a. Holding the attached rope, throw a life belt toward the dog. OR

b. Try to hook the dog's collar with a pole. OR

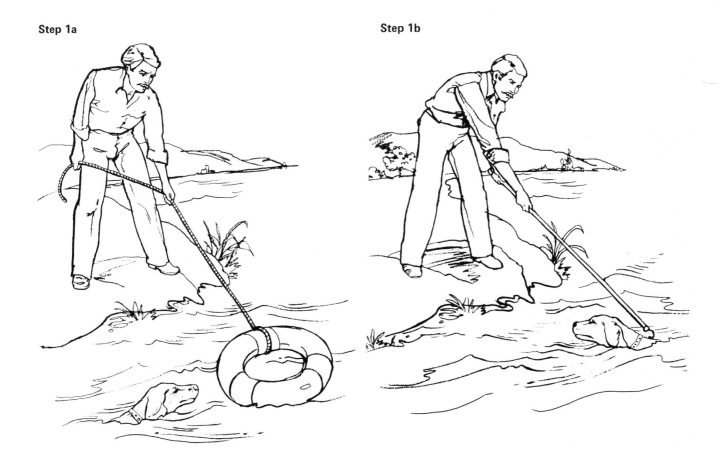

Step 1a

Step 1b

c. Row out to the dog in a boat. OR

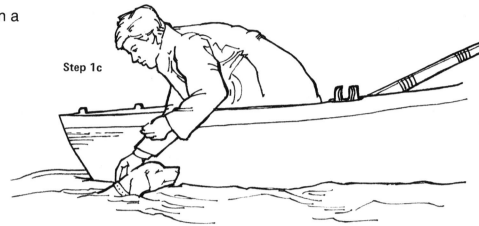

Step 1c

d. As a last resort, swim to the dog. Protect yourself. Bring something for the dog to cling to or climb on and be pulled to shore.

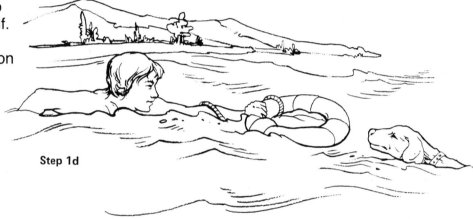

Step 1d

STEP 2: Drain the lungs.

a. If you can lift the dog, grasp the rear legs and hold the animal upside down for 15–20 seconds. Give 3 or 4 downward shakes to help drain fluid from the lungs.

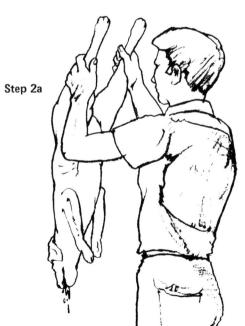

Step 2a

b. If you cannot lift the dog, place it on a sloping surface with its head low to facilitate drainage.

Step 2b

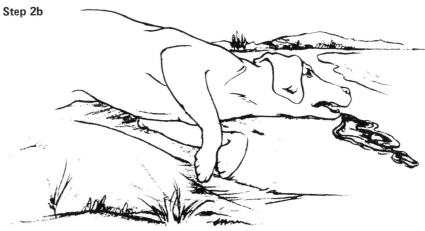

STEP 3: If the dog is not breathing, feel for heartbeat by placing fingers about 2 inches behind the dog's elbow in the middle of its chest.

Step 3

STEP 4: If the heart is not beating, proceed to Step 5. If it is, perform artificial respiration.

a. Turn the dog on its side.

b. Hold the dog's mouth and lips closed and blow firmly into its nostrils. Blow for 3 seconds, take a deep breath, and repeat until you feel resistance or see the chest rise.

Step 4b

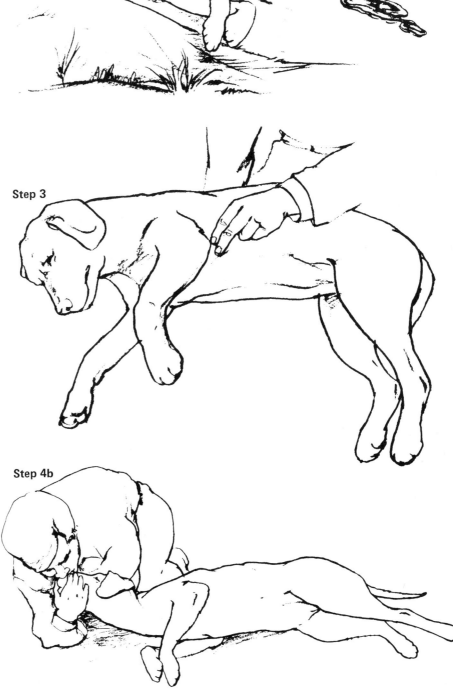

c. After 1 minute, stop. Watch the chest for movement to indicate the dog is breathing on its own.

d. If the dog is not breathing, continue artificial respiration.

STEP 5: If the heart is not beating, perform CPR (cardiopulmonary resuscitation).

CPR for dogs weighing up to 45 pounds

a. Turn the dog on its back.

b. Kneel down at the head of the dog.

c. Clasp your hands over the dog's chest with your palms resting on either side of its chest.

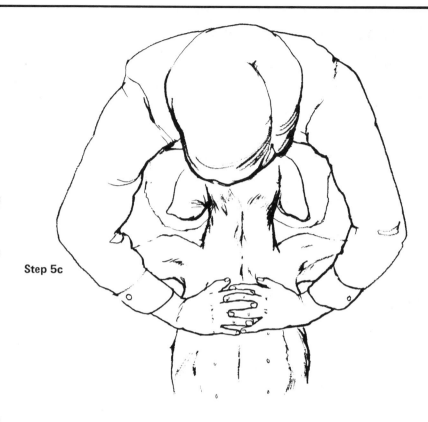

Step 5c

d. Compress your palms on the chest firmly for a count of "2" and release for a count of "1." Moderate pressure is required. Repeat about 30 times in 30 seconds.

e. Alternately (after 30 seconds), hold the dog's mouth and lips closed and blow firmly into its nostrils. Blow for 3 seconds, take a deep breath, and repeat until you feel resistance or see the chest rise. Try to repeat this 20 times in 60 seconds.

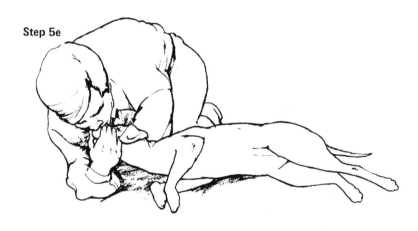

Step 5e

f. After 1 minute, stop. Look at the chest for breathing movement and feel for heartbeat by placing fingers about 2 inches behind the dog's elbow in the centre of its chest.

g. If the dog's heart is not beating, continue CPR. If the heart starts beating, but the dog is still not breathing, return to Step 4.

CPR for dogs weighing over 45 pounds

a. Turn the dog on its side.

b. Place the palm of your hand in the middle of the dog's chest.

c. Press for a count of "2" and release for a count of "1." Firm pressure is required. Repeat about 30 times in 30 seconds.

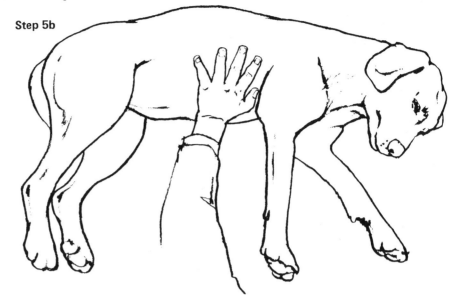

Step 5b

d. Alternately (after 30 seconds), hold the dog's mouth and lips closed and blow firmly into its nostrils. Blow for 3 seconds, take a deep breath, and repeat until you feel resistance or see the chest rise. Try to repeat this 20 times in 60 seconds.

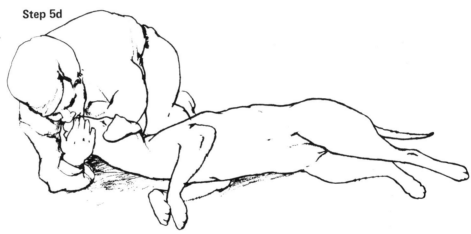

Step 5d

e. After 1 minute, stop. Look at the chest for breathing movement and feel for heartbeat by placing fingers about 2 inches behind the dog's elbow in the centre of its chest.

f. If the dog's heart is not beating, continue CPR. If the heart starts beating, but the dog is still not breathing, return to Step 4.

STEP 6: Contact the veterinary surgeon immediately and take the dog to the surgery. CPR or artificial respiration should be continued on the way to the surgery or until the dog is breathing and its heart is beating without assistance.

Electrical Shock

WATCH FOR SIGNS OF SHOCK:

Pale or white gums, rapid heartbeat and breathing. If signs are present see page 71.

STEP 1: If the dog still has the electric cord in its mouth, DO NOT touch. First remove the plug from its socket.

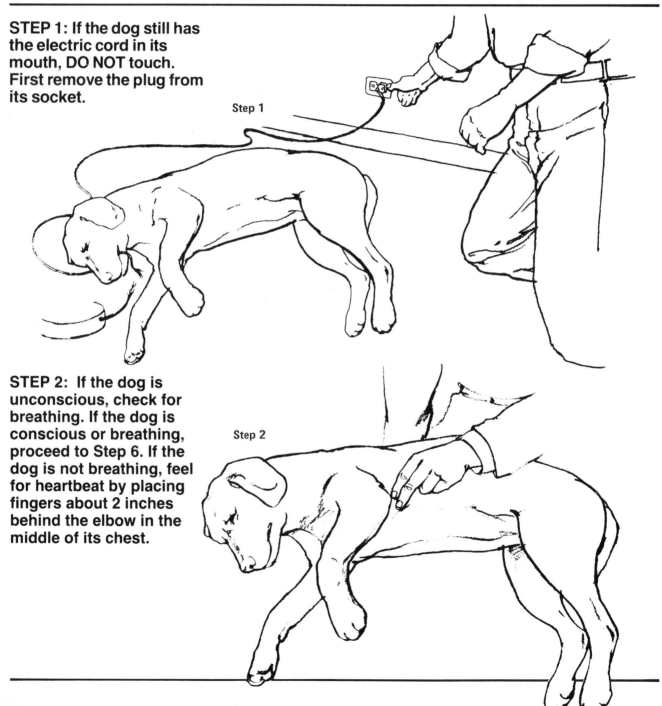

Step 1

STEP 2: If the dog is unconscious, check for breathing. If the dog is conscious or breathing, proceed to Step 6. If the dog is not breathing, feel for heartbeat by placing fingers about 2 inches behind the elbow in the middle of its chest.

Step 2

STEP 3: If the heart is not beating, proceed to Step 4. If it is, perform artificial respiration.

a. Turn the dog on its side.

Step 3b

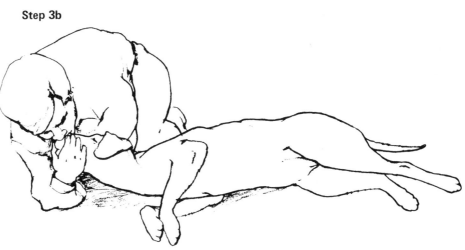

b. Hold the dog's mouth and lips closed and blow firmly into its nostrils. Blow for 3 seconds, take a deep breath, and repeat until you feel resistance or see the chest rise.

c. After 1 minute, stop. Watch the chest for movement to indicate the dog is breathing on its own.

d. If the dog is not breathing, continue artificial respiration.

STEP 4: If the heart is not beating, perform CPR (cardiopulmonary resuscitation).

CPR for dogs weighing up to 45 pounds

a. Turn the dog on its back.

b. Kneel down at the head of the dog.

c. Clasp your hands over the dog's chest with your palms resting on either side of its chest.

Step 4c

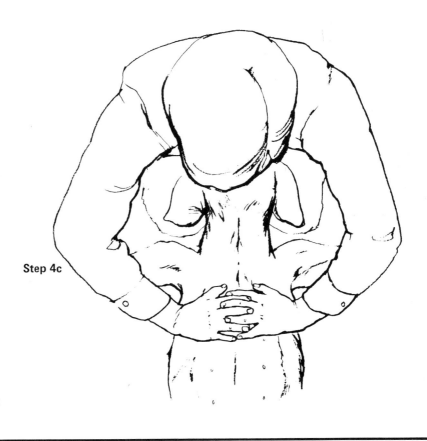

d. Compress your palms on the chest firmly for a count of "2" and release for a count of "1." Moderate pressure is required. Repeat about 30 times in 30 seconds.

e. Alternately (after 30 seconds), hold the dog's mouth and lips closed and blow firmly into its nostrils. Blow for 3 seconds, take a deep breath, and repeat until you feel resistance or see the chest rise. Try to repeat this 20 times in 60 seconds.

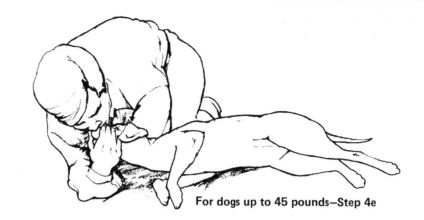

For dogs up to 45 pounds—Step 4e

f. After 1 minute, stop. Look at the chest for breathing movement and feel for heartbeat by placing fingers about 2 inches behind the dog's elbow in the centre of its chest.

g. If the dog's heart is not beating, continue CPR. If the heart starts beating, but the dog is still not breathing, return to Step 3.

CPR for dogs weighing over 45 pounds

a. Turn the dog on its side.

b. Place the palm of your hand in the middle of the dog's chest.

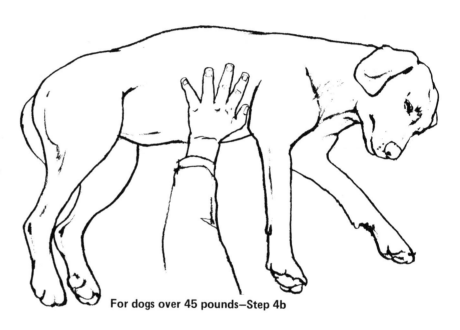

For dogs over 45 pounds—Step 4b

c. Press for a count of "2" and release for a count of "1." Firm pressure is required. Repeat about 30 times in 30 seconds.

d. Alternately (after 30 seconds), hold the dog's mouth and lips closed and blow firmly into its nostrils. Blow for 3 seconds, take a deep breath, and repeat until you feel resistance or see the chest rise. Try to repeat this 20 times in 60 seconds.

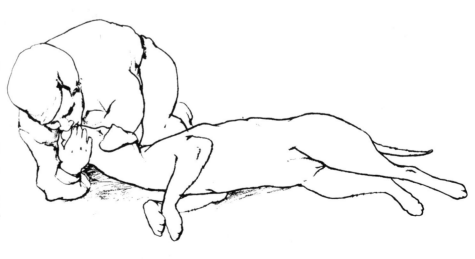

For dogs over 45 pounds—Step 4d

e. After 1 minute, stop. Look at the chest for breathing movement and feel for heartbeat by placing fingers about 2 inches behind the dog's elbow in the centre of its chest.

f. If the dog's heart is not beating, continue CPR. If the heart starts beating, but the dog is still not breathing, return to Step 3.

STEP 5: Telephone the veterinary surgeon and take the dog to the surgery. CPR or artificial respiration should be continued on the way to the surgery or until the dog is breathing and its heart is beating without assistance.

STEP 6: If the dog's mouth or lips are burned (bright red), swab them gently with 3% (10 volumes) hydrogen peroxide.

STEP 7: To conserve body heat, place a hot water bottle (100°F/37°C) against the dog's abdomen. Wrap the bottle in cloth to prevent burns. Wrap the dog in a blanket or jacket.

STEP 8: Telephone the veterinary surgeon and take the dog to the surgery immediately.

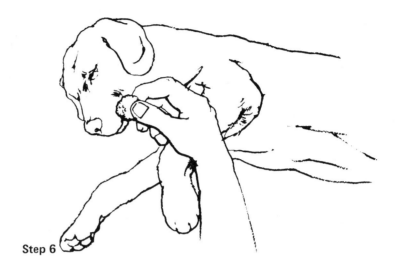

Step 6

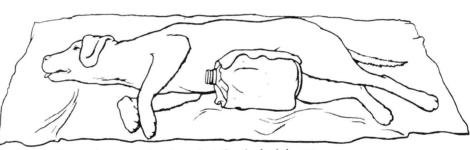

Step 7: Place a hot water bottle against the dog's abdomen.

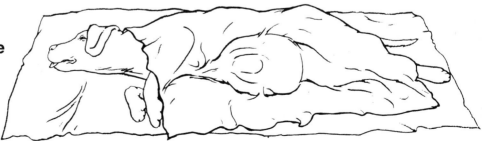

Step 7: Wrap the dog in a blanket or jacket.

Eyeball Out of Socket

| Minutes are important in saving the eye. |

STEP 1: Restrain the dog if necessary. See page 5.

STEP 2: Hold a clean, wet towel over the eye.

STEP 3: Contact the veterinary surgeon and take the dog to the surgery immediately.

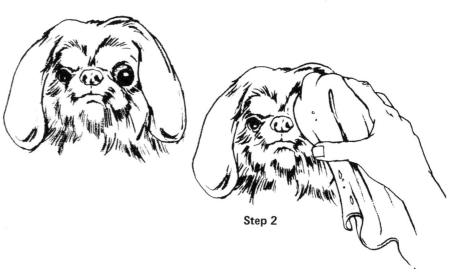

Step 2

Object in Eye

STEP 1: DO NOT try to remove the object.

STEP 2: Restrain the dog if necessary. See page 5.

STEP 3: Prevent self-injury to the eye.

a. Dewclaws (if present) should be bandaged on the front paw on the same side as the affected eye.

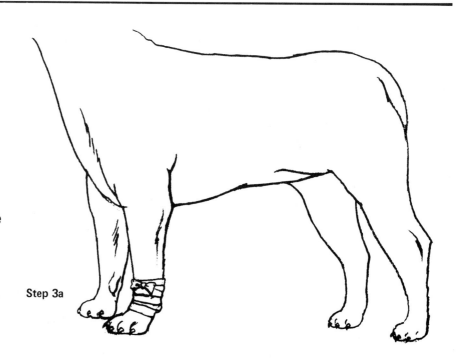

Step 3a

b. For small dogs, cut a piece of large cardboard into an Elizabethan-type collar.

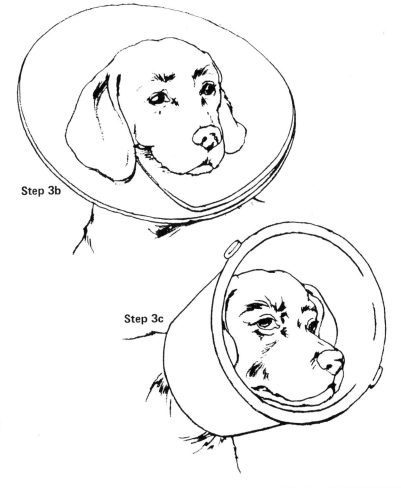

Step 3b

Step 3c

c. For larger dogs, cut the bottom from a plastic bucket, fit the bucket over the dog's head, and hold it in place by tying it to the dog's collar.

STEP 4: Telephone the veterinary surgeon and take the dog to the surgery immediately.

Scratched or Irritated Eye

SIGNS: SQUINTING, RUBBING OR PAWING AT EYES, THICK DISCHARGE OR REDNESS.

STEP 1: Restrain the dog if necessary. See page 5.

STEP 2: Flush thoroughly (3 or 4 times) by pouring plain water into the eye.

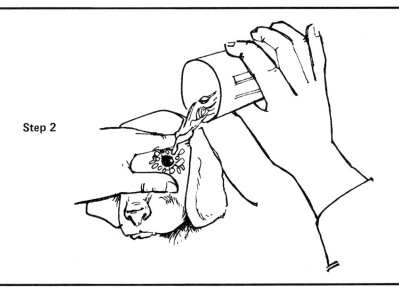

Step 2

STEP 3: Prevent self-injury to the eye.

a. Dewclaws (if present) should be bandaged on the front paw on the same side as the affected eye.

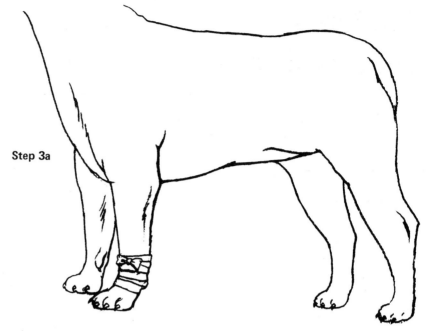

Step 3a

b. For small dogs, cut a piece of large cardboard into an Elizabethan-type collar.

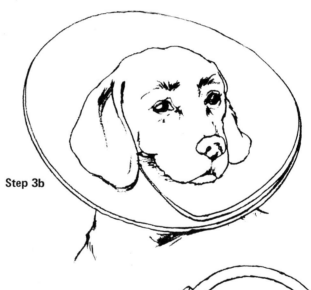

Step 3b

c. For larger dogs, cut the bottom from a plastic bucket, fit the bucket over the dog's head, and hold it in place by tying it to the dog's collar.

STEP 4: Telephone the veterinary surgeon and take the dog to the surgery immediately.

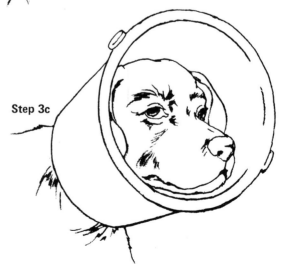

Step 3c

Fish Hook Embedded in Dog

STEP 1: If the hook is in the tongue or roof of the mouth, DO NOT attempt to remove it; take the dog to the veterinary surgeon immediately.

STEP 2: Restrain the dog if necessary. See page 5. If the hook is in the lip, avoid that area when muzzling the dog.

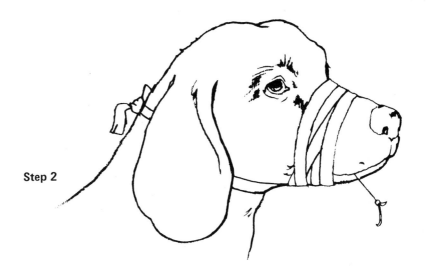

Step 2

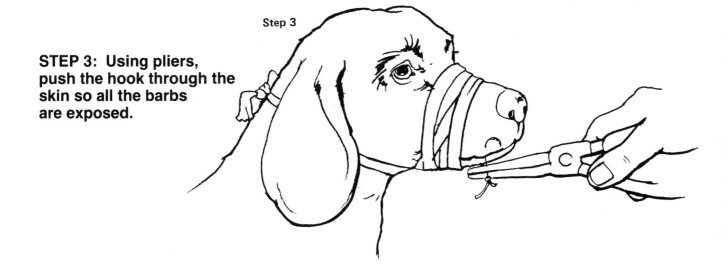

Step 3

STEP 3: Using pliers, push the hook through the skin so all the barbs are exposed.

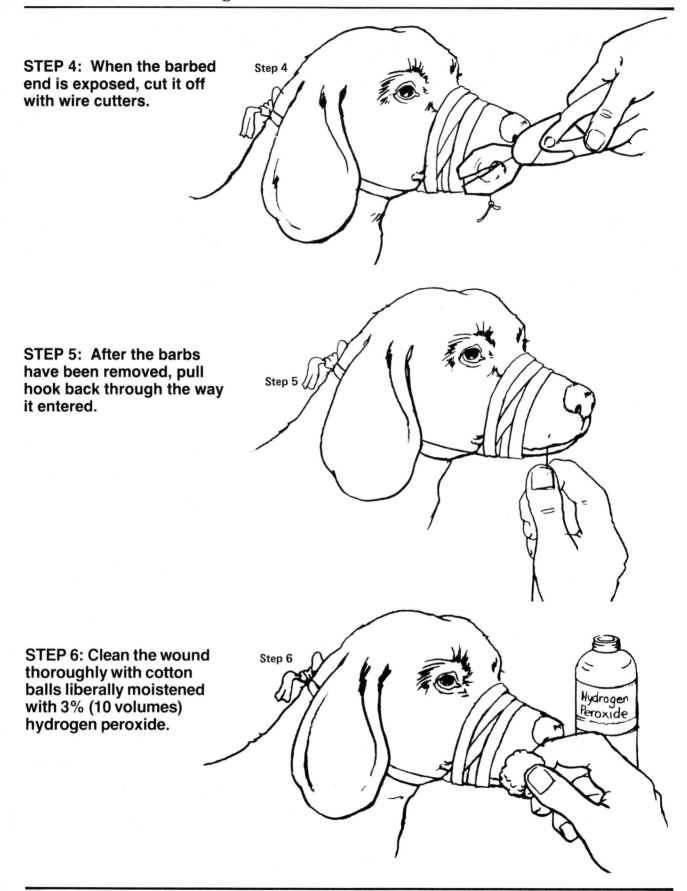

STEP 4: When the barbed end is exposed, cut it off with wire cutters.

Step 4

STEP 5: After the barbs have been removed, pull hook back through the way it entered.

Step 5

STEP 6: Clean the wound thoroughly with cotton balls liberally moistened with 3% (10 volumes) hydrogen peroxide.

Step 6

Hydrogen Peroxide

Frostbite

SIGNS: PAIN, PALE SKIN IN EARLY STAGES, RED OR BLACK SKIN IN ADVANCED STAGES.

The most commonly affected areas are the ears and tail tip.

STEP 1: Restrain the dog if necessary. See page 5.

STEP 2: Warm the area with moist towels. Water temperature should be warm but not hot (75°F/24°C). DO NOT use ointment.

STEP 3: If the skin turns dark, transport to the surgery after contacting the veterinary surgeon.

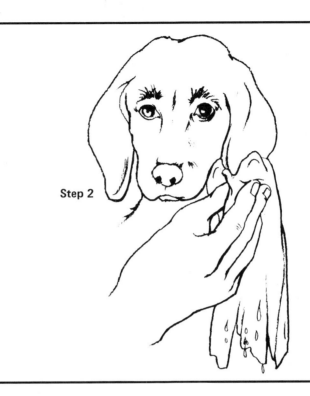

Step 2

Heatstroke

SIGNS: EXCESSIVE DROOLING, LACK OF COORDINATION, RAPID BREATHING, TOP OF THE HEAD HOT TO THE TOUCH.

Prompt treatment is urgent. Heatstroke can lead to brain damage and death.

STEP 1: Remove the dog from the hot environment.

STEP 2: Immerse the dog in a cold water bath or continuously run a garden hose on its body; continue either treatment for at least 30 minutes.

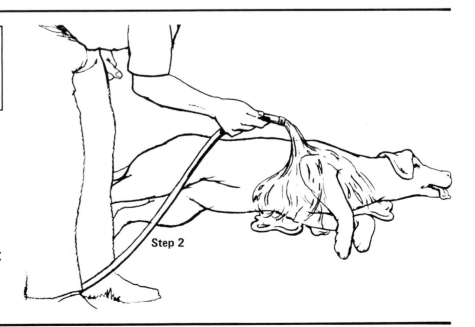

Step 2

STEP 3: Apply ice packs to the top of the head; keep them there while transporting to the veterinary surgeon.

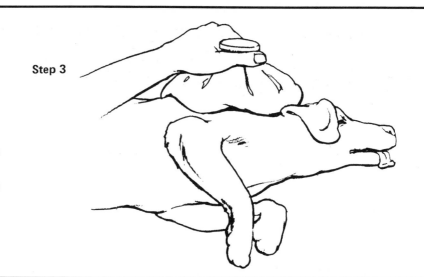

Step 3

STEP 4: Telephone the veterinary surgeon and take the dog to the surgery immediately after the above treatment.

Hypothermia

SIGNS: DEPRESSION, SUBNORMAL BODY TEMPERATURE, COMA.

STEP 1: Warm the dog.

a. Place a hot water bottle (100°F/37°C) against the dog's abdomen. Wrap the bottle in cloth to prevent burns. Wrap the dog in a blanket or jacket. OR

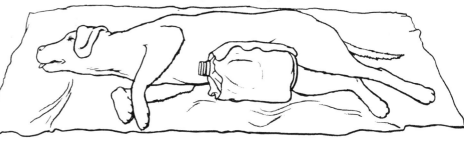

Step 1a: Place a hot water bottle against the dog's abdomen.

b. Use an electric blanket; keep the setting on "low" and turn the dog every few minutes to prevent burns.

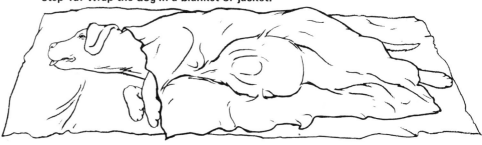

Step 1a: Wrap the dog in a blanket or jacket.

STEP 2: Telephone the veterinary surgeon and take the dog to the surgery immediately.

Insect or Jelly-fish Sting

SIGNS: SWELLING, PAIN IN MUSCLES AND AFFECTED AREA, VOMITING, WEAKNESS, FEVER, SHOCK.

WATCH FOR SIGNS OF SHOCK:

Pale or white gums, rapid heartbeat and breathing. If signs are present see page 71.

Bee, wasp, hornet or jelly-fish stings may produce an allergic reaction.

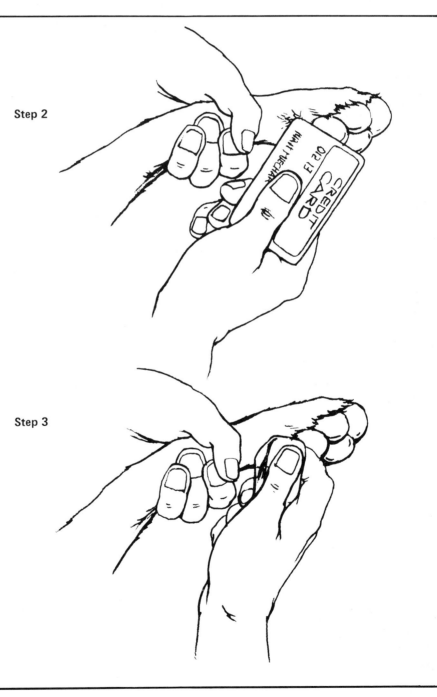

Step 2

Step 3

STEP 1: Restrain the dog if necessary. See page 5.

STEP 2: DO NOT pinch the area. If stung by a bee, scrape the sting off immediately with a credit card or dull knife. Others do not leave the sting in the skin.

STEP 3: Apply ice to the affected area.

STEP 4: Administer any single strength cold tablet or hay fever product that contains an antihistamine, 1 tablet or capsule per 20–25 lbs. body weight.

a. Grasp the dog's upper jaw with one hand over its muzzle.

b. Press the lips over the upper teeth by pressing your thumb on one side and your fingers on the other so that the lips are between its teeth and your fingers. Firm pressure will force the mouth open.

c. Hold the pill between the thumb and index finger of your other hand and place the pill as far back in the mouth as possible.

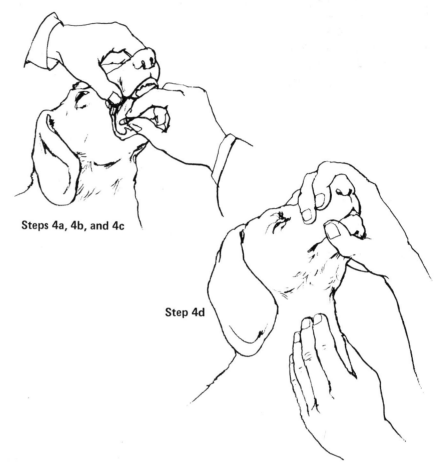

Steps 4a, 4b, and 4c

Step 4d

d. Gently rub the dog's throat to stimulate swallowing.

STEP 5: Telephone the veterinary surgeon and take the dog to the surgery immediately.

Corrosive or Petroleum-Base Poison

SIGNS: BURNS ON MOUTH IF CORROSIVE, CHARACTERISTIC ODOUR IF PETROLEUM PRODUCT, SEVERE ABDOMINAL PAIN, VOMITING, DIARRHOEA, BLOODY URINE, COMA.

WATCH FOR SIGNS OF SHOCK:

Pale or white gums, rapid heartbeat and breathing. If signs are present see page 71.

Corrosives include battery acid, corn and callous remover, dishwasher detergent, drain cleaner, grease remover, lye, oven cleaner. Petroleum products include paint solvent, floor wax, and dry cleaning solution. If in doubt as to type of poison, call the veterinary surgeon.

STEP 1: If the dog is comatose or convulsing, wrap it in a blanket and transport immediately to the veterinary surgeon.

STEP 2: Restrain the dog if necessary. See page 5.

STEP 3: Flush the dog's mouth and muzzle thoroughly with large amounts of water. Hold its head at a slight downward angle so it does not choke.

STEP 4: DO NOT induce vomiting. Give 1 tablespoon of olive oil or egg white.

a. If necessary, apply a mouth-tie loosely to limit jaw movement. See page 6.

b. Tip the dog's head slightly backward.

c. Pull the lower lip out at the corner to make a pouch.

d. Place the fluid slowly into the pouch a little at a time, allowing each small amount to be swallowed before giving any more of the dose.

e. Gently rub the throat to stimulate swallowing.

STEP 5: Take the dog and container of the suspected poison to the veterinary surgeon immediately.

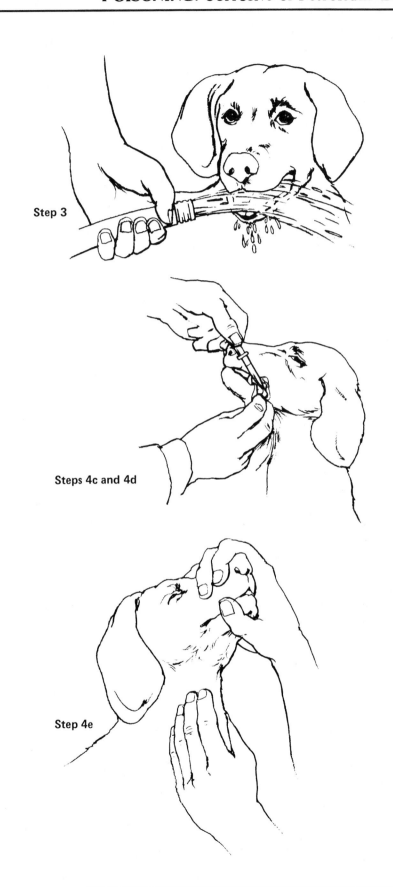

Step 3

Steps 4c and 4d

Step 4e

Noncorrosive Poison

SIGNS: EXCESSIVE DROOLING, VOMITING, ABDOMINAL PAIN, LACK OF COORDINATION.

WATCH FOR SIGNS OF SHOCK: Pale or white gums, rapid heartbeat and breathing. If signs are present see page 71.

STEP 1: Restrain the dog if necessary. See page 5.

STEP 2: If the dog has not already vomited, induce vomiting immediately by giving 1 teaspoon of 3% (10 volumes) hydrogen peroxide per 10 pounds of body weight every 10 minutes until the dog vomits.

a. If necessary, apply a mouth-tie loosely to limit jaw movement. See page 6.

b. Tip the dog's head slightly backward.

c. Pull the lower lip out at the corner to make a pouch.

d. Using a plastic eye dropper or dose syringe, place the fluid slowly into the pouch a little at a time. Allow each small amount to be swallowed before giving any more of the dose.

e. Gently rub the throat to stimulate swallowing.

STEP 3: If no 3% (10 volumes) hydrogen peroxide is available, place a heaped teaspoon of table salt in the back of the dog's mouth every 10 minutes until the dog vomits.

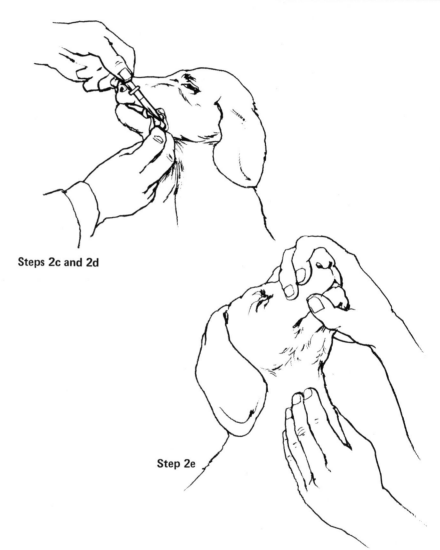

Steps 2c and 2d

Step 2e

a. Grasp the upper jaw with one hand over the muzzle.

b. Press the lips over the upper teeth by pressing your thumb on one side and your fingers on the other so the dog's lips are between its teeth and your fingers. Firm pressure will force the mouth open.

c. Holding the teaspoon of salt in the other hand, place the salt as far back in the mouth as possible.

d. Gently rub the throat to stimulate swallowing.

STEP 4: Save the vomit material for the veterinary surgeon.

STEP 5: Take the dog, vomit, and container of suspected poison to the veterinary surgeon immediately.

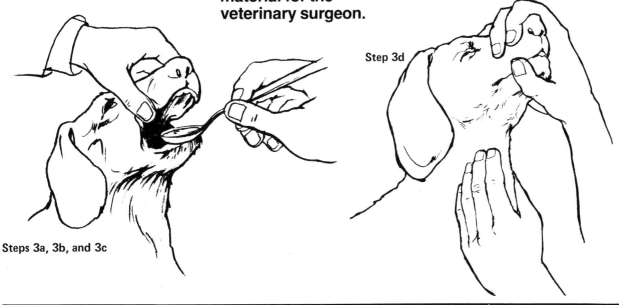

Step 3d

Steps 3a, 3b, and 3c

Poisonous Plants

SIGNS: DROOLING, VOMITING, DIARRHOEA, ABDOMINAL PAIN, INCOORDINATION.

It is safe to assume that all common house plants are toxic to some degree.

STEP 1: Restrain the dog if necessary. See page 5.

STEP 2: If the dog has not already vomited, induce vomiting immediately by giving 1 teaspoon of 3% (10 volumes) hydrogen peroxide per 10 pounds of body weight every 10 minutes until the dog vomits.

a. If necessary, apply a mouth-tie loosely to limit jaw movement. See page 6.

b. Tip the dog's head slightly backward.

c. Pull the lower lip out at the corner to make a pouch.

d. Using a plastic eye dropper or dose syringe, place the fluid slowly into the pouch a little at a time. Allow each small amount to be swallowed before giving any more of the dose.

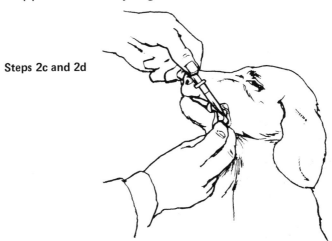

Steps 2c and 2d

e. Gently rub the throat to stimulate swallowing.

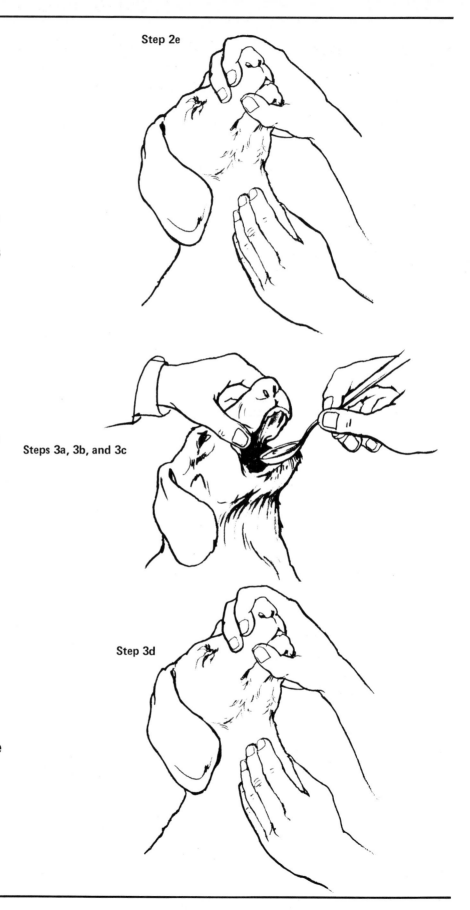

Step 2e

STEP 3: If no 3% (10 volumes) hydrogen peroxide is available, place a heaped teaspoon of table salt in the back of the dog's mouth every 10 minutes until the dog vomits.

a. Grasp the upper jaw with one hand over the muzzle.

b. Press the lips over the upper teeth by pressing your thumb on one side and your fingers on the other so the dog's lips are between its teeth and your fingers. Firm pressure will force the mouth open.

Steps 3a, 3b, and 3c

c. Holding the teaspoon of salt in the other hand, place the salt as far back in the mouth as possible.

d. Gently rub the throat to stimulate swallowing.

Step 3d

STEP 4: If convulsions or difficulty in breathing develops, telephone the veterinary surgeon and take the dog and a leaf of the suspected plant to the surgery immediately.

Smoke or Carbon Monoxide Inhalation

SIGNS: DEPRESSION, LACK OF COORDINATION, HEAVY PANTING, DEEP RED GUMS, POSSIBLE CONVULSIONS.

WATCH FOR SIGNS OF SHOCK:

Pale or white gums, rapid heartbeat and breathing. If signs are present see page 71.

A. If conscious

STEP 1: Remove the dog to fresh air immediately.

STEP 2: Flush the dog's eyes thoroughly by pouring plain water directly into them.

STEP 3: Contact the veterinary surgeon and take the dog to the surgery immediately.

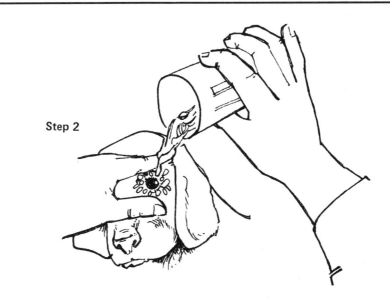

Step 2

B. If unconscious

STEP 1: Remove the dog to fresh air immediately.

STEP 2: If the dog is not breathing, feel for heartbeat by placing fingers about 2 inches behind the dog's elbow in the middle of its chest.

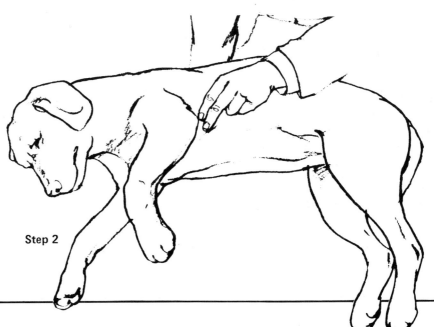

Step 2

STEP 3: If the heart is not beating, proceed to Step 4. If it is, perform artificial respiration.

a. Turn the dog on its side.

b. Hold the dog's mouth and lips closed and blow firmly into its nostrils. Blow for 3 seconds, take a deep breath, and repeat until you feel resistance or see the chest rise.

c. After 1 minute, stop. Watch the chest for movement to indicate the dog is breathing on its own.

d. If the dog is not breathing, continue artificial respiration.

STEP 4: If the heart is not beating, perform CPR (cardiopulmonary resuscitation).

CPR for dogs weighing up to 45 pounds

a. Turn the dog on its back.

b. Kneel down at the head of the dog.

c. Clasp your hands over the dog's chest with your palms resting on either side of its chest.

d. Compress your palms on the chest firmly for a count of "2" and release for a count of "1." Moderate pressure is required. Repeat about 30 times in 30 seconds.

e. Alternately (after 30 seconds), hold the dog's mouth and lips closed and blow firmly into its nostrils.

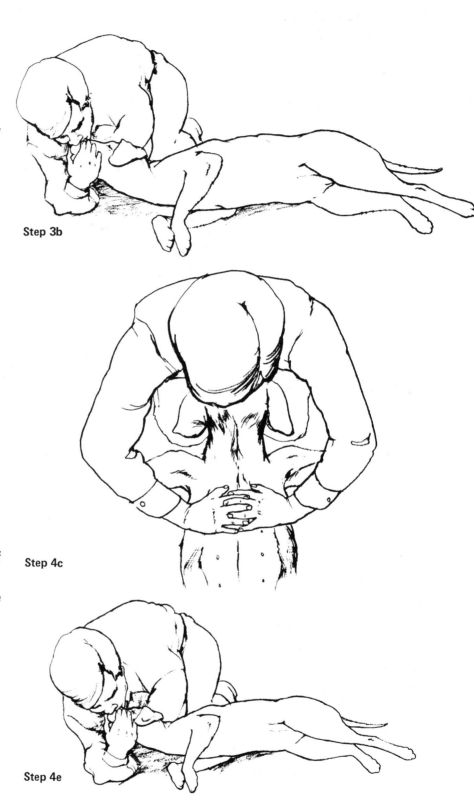

Step 3b

Step 4c

Step 4e

Blow for 3 seconds, take a deep breath, and repeat until you feel resistance or see the chest rise. Try to repeat this 20 times in 60 seconds.

f. After 1 minute, stop. Look at the chest for breathing movement and feel for heartbeat by placing fingers about 2 inches behind the dog's elbow in the centre of its chest.

g. If the dog's heart is not beating, continue CPR. If the heart starts beating, breathing, return to Step 3.

CPR for dogs weighing over 45 pounds

a. Turn the dog on its side.

b. Place the palm of your hand in the middle of the dog's chest.

c. Press for a count of "2" and release for a count of "1." Firm pressure is required. Repeat about 30 times in 30 seconds.

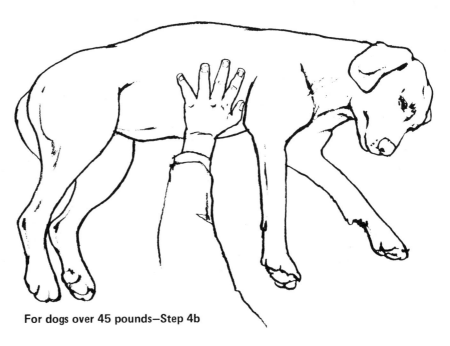

For dogs over 45 pounds—Step 4b

d. Alternately (after 30 seconds), hold the dog's mouth and lips closed and blow firmly into its nostrils. Blow for 3 seconds, take a deep breath, and repeat until you feel resistance or see the chest rise. Try to repeat this 20 times in 60 seconds.

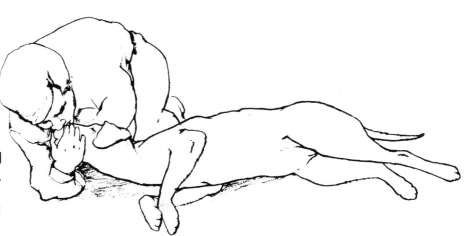

For dogs over 45 pounds—Step 4d

e. After 1 minute, stop. Look at the chest for breathing movement and feel for heartbeat by placing fingers about 2 inches behind the dog's elbow in the centre of its chest.

f. If the dog's heart is not beating, continue CPR. If the heart starts beating, but the dog is still not breathing, return to Step 3.

STEP 5: Telephone the veterinary surgeon. CPR or artificial respiration should be continued on the way to the surgery or until the dog is breathing and its heart is beating without assistance.

Porcupine Quills

Porcupines do not occur in Great Britain. Readers visiting countries where they live will find the treatment useful.

STEP 1: Restrain the dog if necessary. See page 5. Avoid quills when tying the mouth shut.

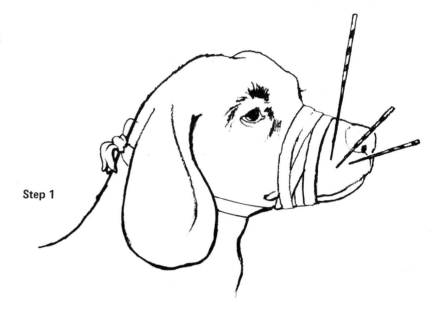

Step 1

STEP 2: Clamp pliers around the quill, as close to skin as possible. Slowly twist and pull straight out.

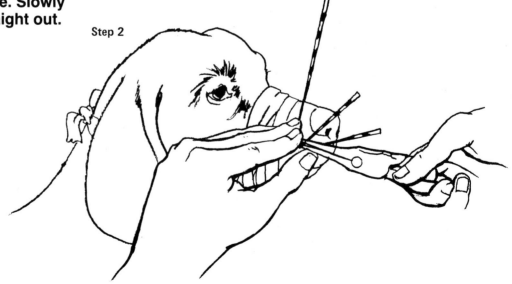

Step 2

STEP 3: To conserve body heat and prevent shock, place a hot water bottle (100°F/37°C) against the dog's abdomen. Wrap the bottle in cloth to prevent burns. Wrap the dog in a blanket or jacket.

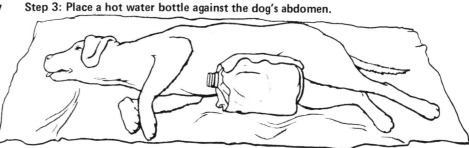
Step 3: Place a hot water bottle against the dog's abdomen.

STEP 4: Transport immediately to the surgery after telephoning the veterinary surgeon.

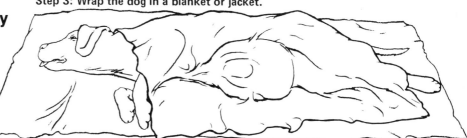
Step 3: Wrap the dog in a blanket or jacket.

Puncture Wound

WATCH FOR SIGNS OF SHOCK: Pale or white gums, rapid heartbeat and breathing. If signs are present see page 71.

A. If the object (knife, arrow, stick, etc.) is protruding

STEP 1: Restrain the dog if necessary, taking care not to touch the object. See page 5.

STEP 2: DO NOT attempt to remove the object.

STEP 3: Place a clean cloth or sterile dressing around the point of entry.

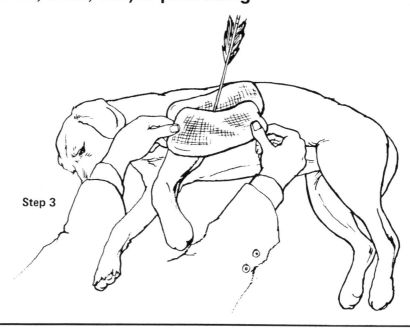
Step 3

STEP 4: Bandage tightly around the point of entry.

STEP 5: Telephone the veterinary surgeon and take the dog to the surgery immediately.

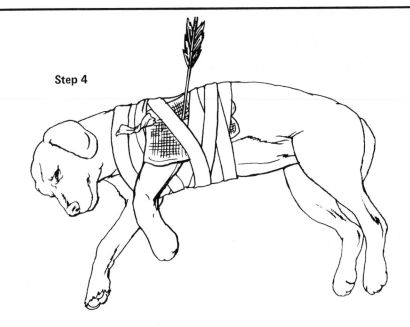

Step 4

B. Other puncture wounds

STEP 1: Restrain the dog if necessary. See page 5.

STEP 2: If the wound is in the chest and a "sucking" noise is heard, bandage tightly enough to seal the wound and after telephoning the veterinary surgeon, take the dog to the surgery immediately.

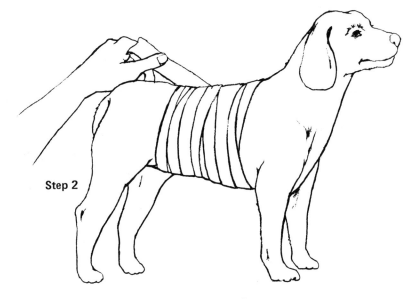

Step 2

STEP 3: Clip the hair around the wound.

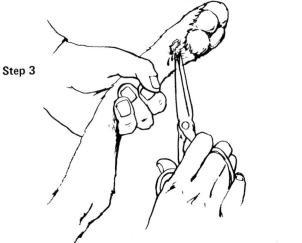

Step 3

STEP 4: Examine the wound carefully for foreign objects such as glass or wood splinters. If present, remove with tweezers or needle-nose pliers.

STEP 5: Flush thoroughly by pouring 3% (10 volumes) hydrogen peroxide or weak salt solution (1 teaspoon of salt to 1 pint of water) into the wound. DO NOT use any other antiseptic.

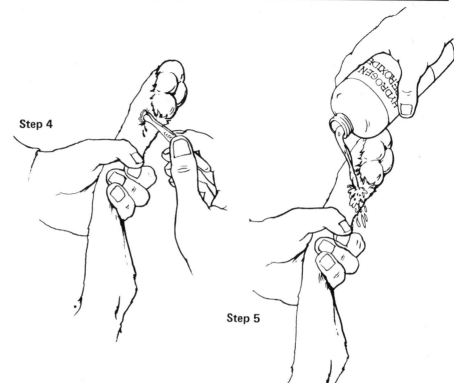

Step 4

Step 5

STEP 6: DO NOT bandage. Allow the wound to drain unless there is excessive bleeding. If the wound DOES bleed excessively:

a. Cover the wound with a clean cloth or sterile dressing.

b. Place your hand over the dressing and press firmly.

c. Keep pressure on the dressing to stop bleeding. If blood soaks through the dressing, DO NOT remove. Apply more dressing and continue to apply pressure until bleeding stops. If bleeding does not stop within 5 minutes, proceed to Step 7.

d. Wrap torn rags or other soft material around the dressing and tie or tape just tightly enough to keep the bandage in place.

Step 6a: Stop bleeding only if the wound bleeds excessively.

Step 6d

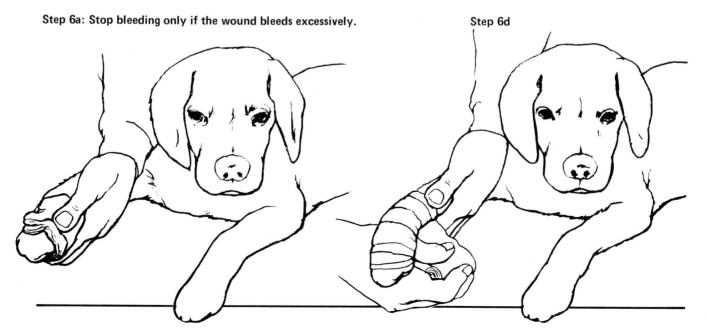

STEP 7: If bleeding does not stop within 5 minutes, apply a tourniquet. DO NOT apply a tourniquet to the head or torso.

a. Use a tie, belt, or piece of cloth folded to about one inch width. DO NOT use rope, wire, or string.

b. Place the material between the wound and the heart, an inch or two above, but not touching, the wound.

Step 7b

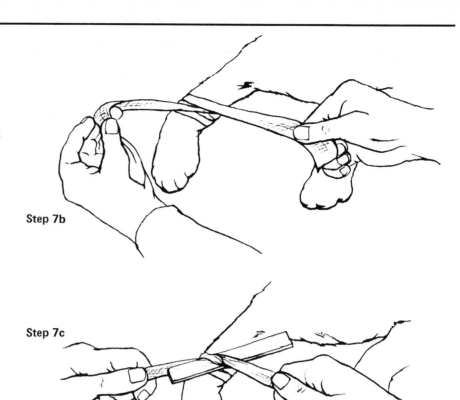

Step 7c

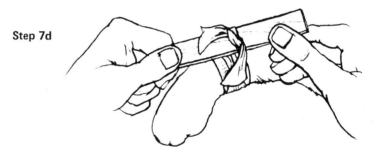

c. Tie a stick or ruler to the material with a single knot.

d. Twist the stick until bleeding stops, but no tighter.

Step 7d

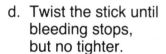

e. Wrap a piece of cloth around the stick and limb to keep in place.

Step 7e

STEP 8: If it will take time to reach the veterinary surgeon, loosen the tourniquet every 15 minutes for a period of 1-2 minutes and then tighten again.

STEP 9: Telephone the veterinary surgeon and take the dog to the surgery.

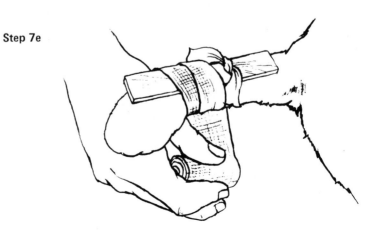

Shock

SIGNS: PALE OR WHITE GUMS, VERY FAST HEARTBEAT (OVER 150 BEATS PER MINUTE), RAPID BREATHING.

Any trauma or serious injury can cause shock. If the dog is in shock, do not take time to splint fractures or treat minor injuries.

STEP 1: Examine for shock.

a. Examine the gums by gently lifting the upper lip so the gum is visible. Pale or white gums indicate the dog is almost certainly in shock and may have serious internal injuries and/or bleeding. If the gums are pink the dog is probably not in shock.

b. Determine the heartbeat. Place fingers firmly on the dog's chest about 2 inches behind the dog's elbow in the centre of its chest. Count the number of beats in 10 seconds and multiply by 6. If the dog is in shock its heartbeat may be over 150 beats per minute.

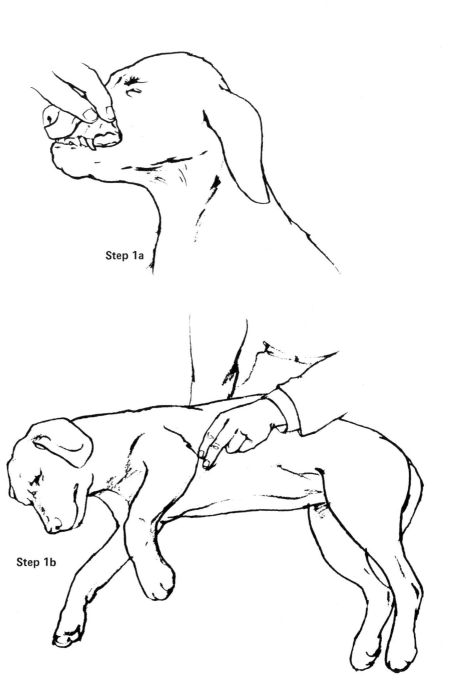

Step 1a

Step 1b

STEP 2: Place dog on its side with its head extended.

STEP 3: Gently pull out the dog's tongue to keep the airway open.

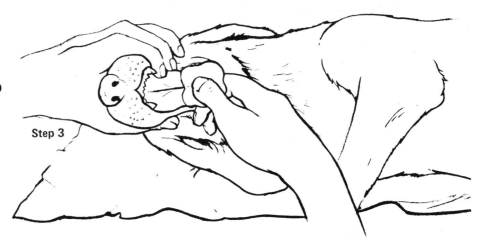

Step 3

STEP 4: Elevate the dog's hindquarters slightly by placing them on a pillow or folded towels.

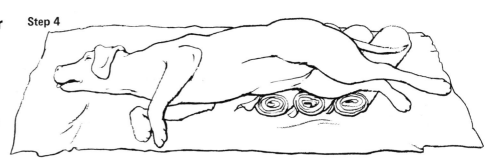

Step 4

STEP 5: Stop visible bleeding immediately; if blood is spurting and the wound is on the leg or tail, proceed to Step 6. If there is no visible bleeding proceed to Step 8.

a. Cover the wound with a clean cloth or sterile dressing.

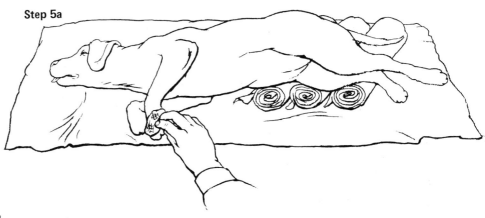

Step 5a

b. Place your hand over the dressing and press firmly.

c. Keep pressure on the dressing to stop bleeding. If blood soaks through the dressing, DO NOT remove. Apply more dressing and continue to apply pressure until bleeding stops. If bleeding does not stop within 5 minutes, proceed to Step 6.

d. Wrap torn rags or other soft material around the dressing and tie or tape just tightly enough to keep the bandage in place.

STEP 6: If bleeding does not stop within 5 minutes or if blood is spurting, apply a tourniquet. DO NOT apply a tourniquet to the head or torso.

a. Use a tie, belt, or piece of cloth folded to about one inch width. DO NOT use rope, wire, or string.

b. Place the material between the wound and the heart, an inch or two above, but not touching, the wound.

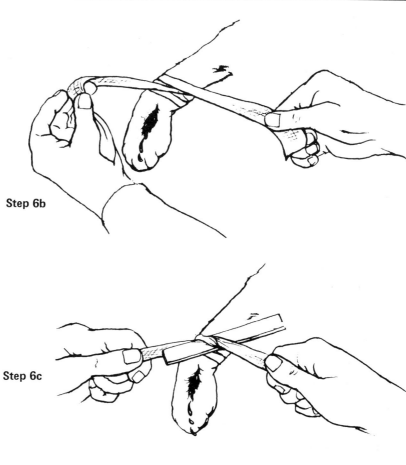

Step 6b

c. Tie a stick or ruler to the material with a single knot.

Step 6c

d. Twist the stick until bleeding stops, but no tighter.

Step 6d

e. Wrap a piece of cloth around the stick and limb to keep in place.

Step 6e

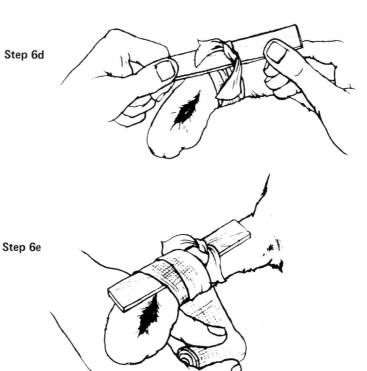

STEP 7: If it will take time to reach the veterinary surgeon, loosen the tourniquet every 15 minutes for a period of 1-2 minutes and then tighten again.

Step 8: Place a hot water bottle against the dog's abdomen.

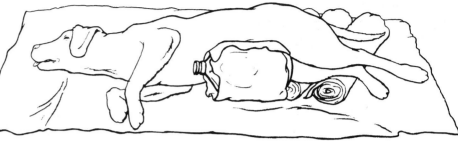

STEP 8: To conserve body heat, place a hot water bottle (100°F/37°C) against the abdomen. Wrap the bottle in cloth to prevent burns. Wrap the dog in a blanket or jacket.

STEP 9: Telephone the veterinary surgeon and take the dog to the surgery immediately.

Step 8: Wrap the dog in a blanket or jacket.

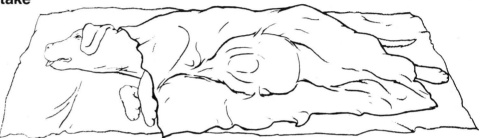

Skin Conditions: Acute Moist Eczema

Acute moist eczema can appear very rapidly, following a wound, skin parasites, contact with an irritant chemical or other causes. Any area of the body covered by thick hair can be affected.

STEP 1: Restrain the dog and if necessary apply a muzzle, as the condition can be painful.

STEP 2: Clip hair from moist red areas of skin.

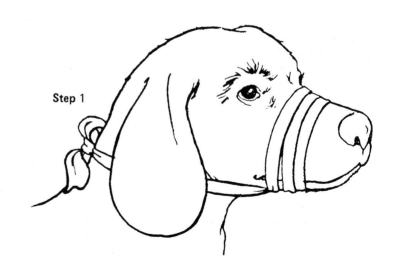

Step 1

STEP 3: Clean area with 3% (10 volumes) hydrogen peroxide or weak salt solution (1 teaspoon of salt to 1 pint of water) and dry with cotton wool.

STEP 4: Apply an antihistamine cream sparingly to the inflamed skin.

STEP 5: Eliminate any skin parasites using an insecticidal spray or powder.

STEP 6: Consult your veterinary surgeon if there is no improvement within 24 hours.

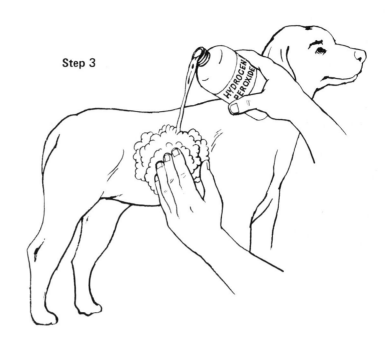

Step 3

Poisonous Snakebite

SIGNS: TWO FANG MARKS, PAIN, SWELLING, VOMITING, DIFFICULTY IN BREATHING, POSSIBLE PARALYSIS AND CONVULSIONS.

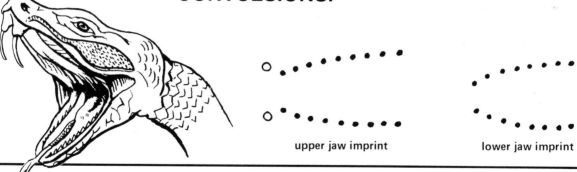

upper jaw imprint   lower jaw imprint

WATCH FOR SIGNS OF SHOCK: Pale or white gums, rapid heartbeat and breathing. If signs are present see page 71.

Treatment must begin as soon as possible after the bite. The adder is the only poisonous snake in Great Britain and is identified by black zigzag markings along the body.

STEP 1: Restrain the dog if necessary. See page 5. Keep exercise to a minimum. Proceed to Step 2 only if there is a delay in obtaining veterinary treatment.

STEP 2: If the bite is on head or torso, proceed to Step 3. If bite is on tail or leg, apply a tourniquet.

a. Use a tie, belt, or piece of cloth folded to about one inch width.

b. Place the material between the bite and heart, an inch or two above, but not touching, the bite.

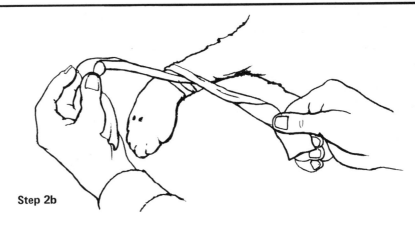

Step 2b

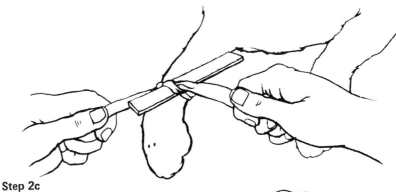

c. Tie a stick or ruler to the material with a single knot.

Step 2c

d. Twist the stick just tightly enough to cut off circulation to the bite area.

Step 2d

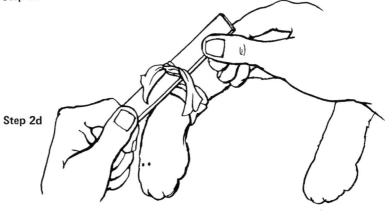

e. Wrap a piece of cloth around the stick and limb to keep in place.

Step 2e

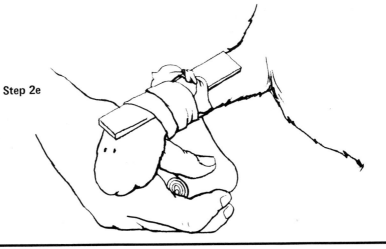

STEP 3: Clip the hair from the bite area.

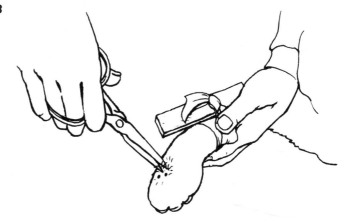

Step 3

CAUTION: Do not use this technique if you have open sores or cuts on your lips, tongue, or inside cheeks; the poison can be absorbed into your system.

STEP 4: Use your mouth to suck venom out of the area. Use heavy suction and repeat several times. Spit out the blood; DO NOT swallow it.

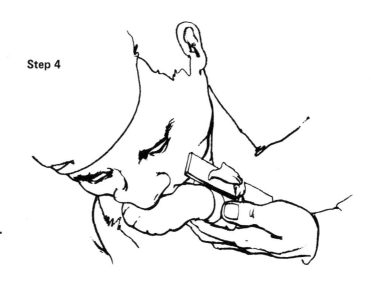

Step 4

STEP 5: Flush thoroughly by pouring 3% (10 volumes) hydrogen peroxide directly on the bite.

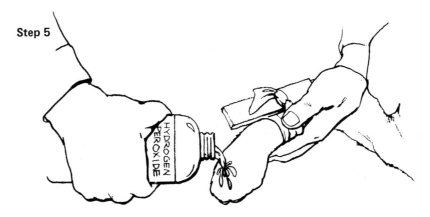

Step 5

STEP 6: Apply ice to the bite area.

STEP 7: If it will take time to reach the veterinary surgeon, loosen the tourniquet every 15 minutes for a period of just 10 seconds, then retighten.

STEP 8: Transport immediately to the veterinary surgeon.

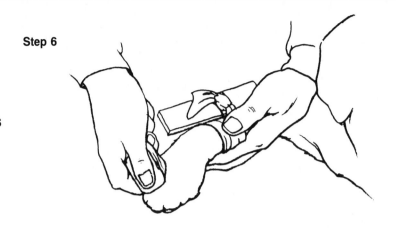

Step 6

Nonpoisonous Snakebite

SIGNS: "U"-SHAPED BITE, PAIN IN BITE AREA.

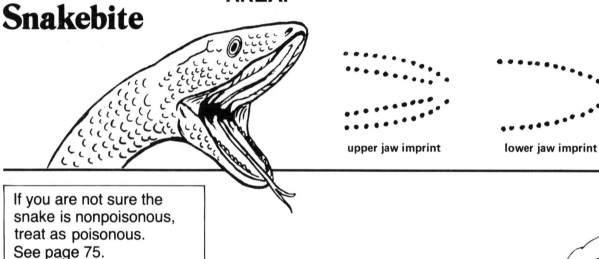

upper jaw imprint   lower jaw imprint

If you are not sure the snake is nonpoisonous, treat as poisonous. See page 75.

STEP 1: Restrain the dog if necessary. See page 5.

STEP 2: Clip the hair from the bite area.

STEP 3: Flush thoroughly by pouring 3% (10 volumes) hydrogen peroxide directly on the bite.

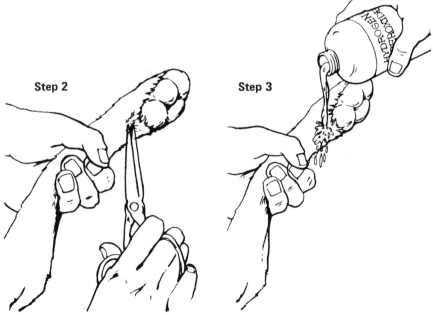

Step 2   Step 3

Toad Poisoning

SIGNS: EXCESSIVE DROOLING, SHAKING HEAD, TREMBLING AND SHAKING BODY, LACK OF COORDINATION, DIFFICULTY BREATHING, CONVULSIONS, COMA.

WATCH FOR SIGNS OF SHOCK:

Pale or white gums, rapid heartbeat and breathing. If signs are present see page 71.

Signs develop immediately after contact of the toad (Bufo species) with the mouth or eyes of the dog.

STEP 1: Restrain the dog if necessary. See page 5.

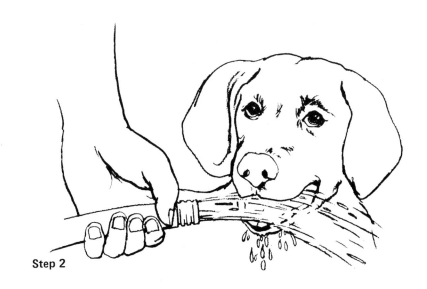

Step 2

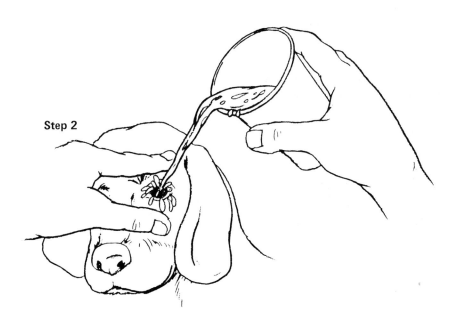

Step 2

STEP 2: Flush the dog's mouth and eyes thoroughly with water, being careful not to choke it. Keep its head tilted at a slight downward angle.

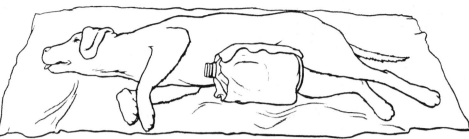

Step 3: Place a hot water bottle against the dog's abdomen.

STEP 3: If the dog is unconscious, place a hot water bottle (100°F/37°C) against its abdomen. Wrap the bottle in cloth to prevent burns. Wrap the dog in a blanket or jacket.

STEP 4: Contact the veterinary surgeon and take the dog to the surgery immediately.

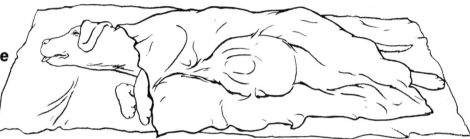

Step 3: Wrap the dog in a blanket or jacket.

Unconsciousness

STEP 1: If you suspect choking, see page 36.

STEP 2: If the dog is breathing, check for shock. See page 71. If the dog is not breathing, proceed to Step 3.

STEP 3: Feel for heartbeat by placing fingers about 2 inches behind the dog's elbow in the middle of its chest.

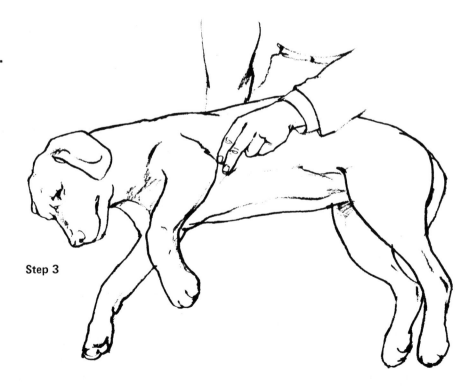

Step 3

STEP 4: If the heart is not beating, proceed to Step 5. If it is, perform artificial respiration.

a. Turn the dog on its side.

b. Hold the dog's mouth and lips closed and blow firmly into its nostrils. Blow for 3 seconds, take a deep breath, and repeat until you feel resistance or see the chest rise.

c. After 1 minute, stop. Watch the chest for movement to indicate the dog is breathing on its own.

d. If the dog is not breathing, continue artificial respiration.

STEP 5: If the heart is not beating, perform CPR (cardiopulmonary resuscitation).

CPR for dogs weighing up to 45 pounds

a. Turn the dog on its back.

b. Kneel down at the head of the dog.

c. Clasp your hands over the dog's chest with your palms resting on either side of its chest.

d. Compress your palms on the chest firmly for a count of "2" and release for a count of "1." Moderate pressure is required. Repeat about 30 times in 30 seconds.

e. Alternately (after 30 seconds), hold the dog's mouth and lips closed and blow firmly into its nostrils. Blow for 3 seconds, take a deep breath, and repeat

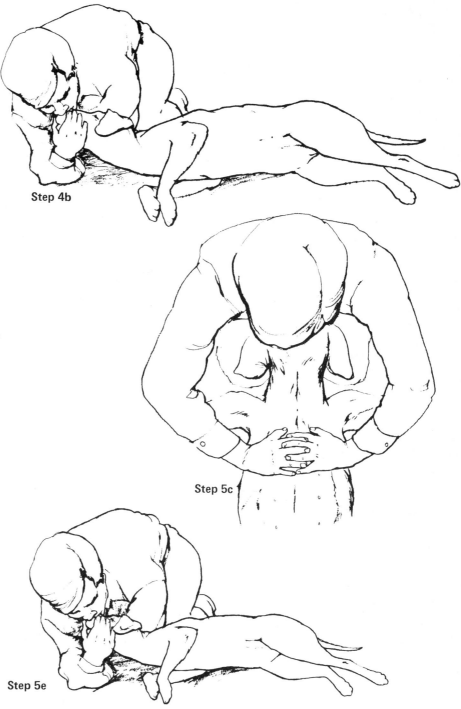

Step 4b

Step 5c

Step 5e

until you feel resistance or see the chest rise. Try to repeat this 20 times in 60 seconds.

f. After 1 minute, stop. Look at the chest for breathing movement and feel for heartbeat by placing

fingers about 2 inches behind the dog's elbow in the centre of its chest.

g. If the dog's heart is not beating, continue CPR. If the heart starts beating, but the dog is still not breathing, return to Step 4.

CPR for dogs weighing over 45 pounds

a. Turn the dog on its side.

b. Place the palm of your hand in the middle of the dog's chest.

c. Press for a count of "2" and release for a count of "1." Firm pressure is required. Repeat about 30 times in 30 seconds.

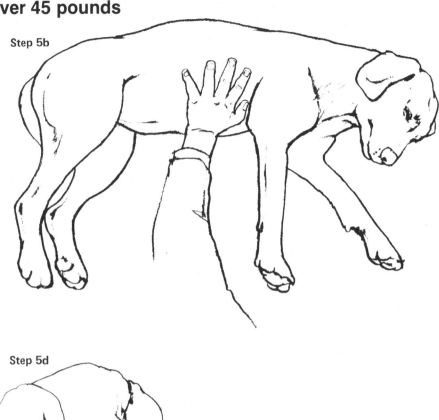

Step 5b

d. Alternately (after 30 seconds), hold the dog's mouth and lips closed and blow firmly into its nostrils. Blow for 3 seconds, take a deep breath, and repeat until you feel resistance or see the chest rise. Try to repeat this 20 times in 60 seconds.

Step 5d

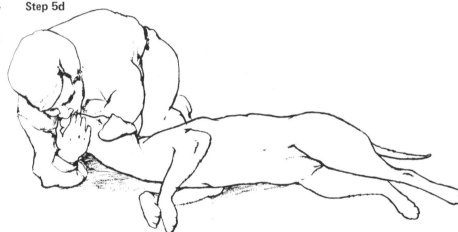

e. After 1 minute, stop. Look at the chest for breathing movement and feel for heartbeat by placing fingers about 2 inches behind the dog's elbow in the centre of its chest.

f. If the dog's heart is not beating, continue CPR. If the heart starts beating, but the dog is still not breathing, return to Step 4.

STEP 6: Telephone the veterinary surgeon immediately. CPR or artificial respiration should be continued on the way to the surgery or until the dog is breathing and its heart is beating without assistance.

Vomiting

STEP 1: Remove all food and water immediately.

STEP 2: If vomiting contains blood or is frequent, contact the veterinary surgeon immediately. If not proceed to Step 3.

STEP 3: Treat with Pepto-Bismol every 4 hours at the rate of 1 teaspoon per 10-15 pounds of the dog's weight. See ADMINISTERING ORAL MEDICINE, page 13.

STEP 4: DO NOT attempt to feed or give water for at least 12 hours.

STEP 5: After 12 hours, feed the dog a mixture of small quantities of boiled minced beef or mutton, cooked rice, and cottage cheese. If this is held down, a transition to regular diet should take place over the next 2 days by mixing an increasing quantity of regular dog food with the minced beef or mutton.

Whelping Problems

Any of the following requires immediate veterinary care:

a. Failure to deliver within 3 hours of intermittent labour.

b. Failure to deliver within 30 minutes of continuous hard labour.

c. Heavy bright red bleeding during labour.

d. Brown or foul-smelling discharge during labour.

e. General weakness of the bitch.

f. Failure to deliver by the 65th day.

g. Presentation of the first water sac with no delivery after 1 hour.

A. If the puppy is stuck in the birth canal with half of its body exposed

STEP 1: Grasp the puppy with a clean towel.

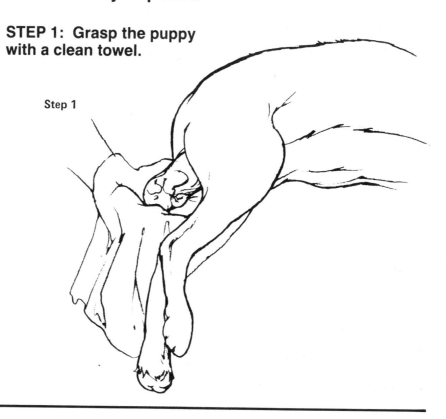

Step 1

STEP 2: Applying steady traction, gently pull the puppy at a slight downward angle. Continue pulling gently and steadily until the pup is delivered.

STEP 3: If you are unable to remove the puppy, contact the veterinary surgeon immediately.

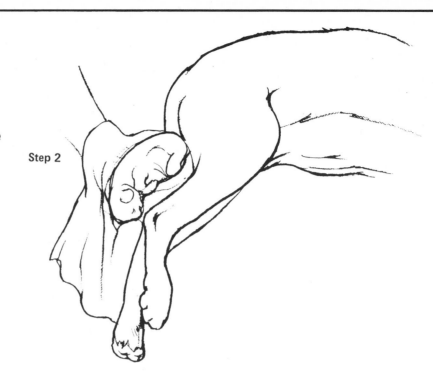

Step 2

B. If, after delivery, the puppy is not cleaned immediately by the bitch

STEP 1: Put the pup, covered in the foetal membrane, into a clean towel.

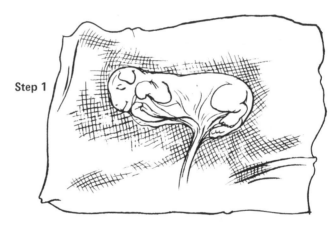

Step 1

STEP 2: Peel the membrane off its face immediately.

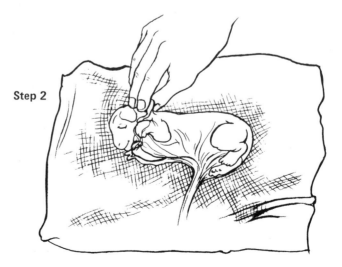

Step 2

STEP 3: Continue to pull the membrane from its body. The membrane will collect around the umbilical cord. DO NOT pull on the umbilical cord.

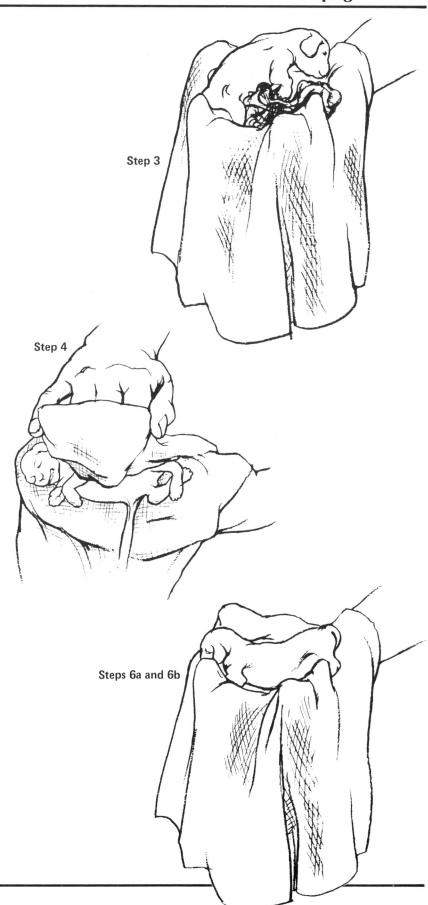

Step 3

STEP 4: Wipe any fluid off the nostrils and mouth. Rub the puppy's body vigorously with a towel to stimulate breathing.

Step 4

STEP 5: If there is heavy mucus in the mouth and nose, clean out what you can with your finger.

STEP 6: If the puppy is still having trouble breathing:

a. Place the puppy in a towel on the palm of your hand.

b. Cradle its head by closing your thumb toward your fingers.

Steps 6a and 6b

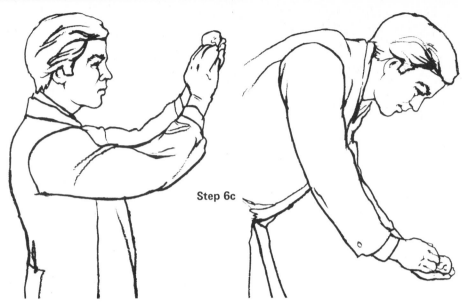

Step 6c

c. Using your other hand to secure the puppy, lift your hands to head level and swing firmly down toward the floor. Repeat several times.

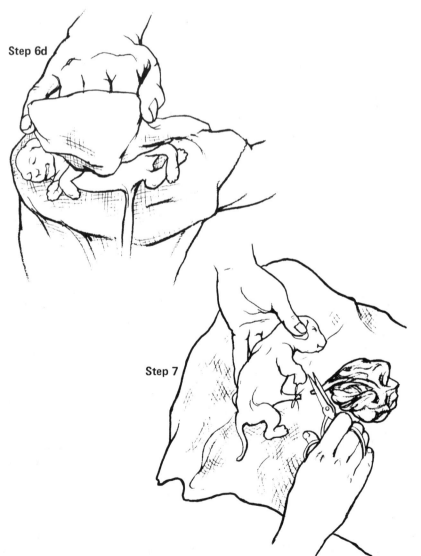

Step 6d

d. Vigorously rub the puppy again with the towel.

e. Stop when the puppy is actively moving and crying.

STEP 7: Tie a thread around the umbilical cord about 1 inch above the puppy's abdomen. Leaving the tied portion attached to the puppy, cut off the rest of the umbilical cord and foetal membrane.

STEP 8: Place the puppy with its mother. She will take care of the rest. If she does not take care of the puppies, or if any other problem develops, contact the veterinary surgeon as soon as possible.

Step 7

The Whys of Emergency Treatment

Restraining an Injured Dog

If the dog is conscious, you must get close enough to it to look it over carefully. But an injured dog is usually frightened and in pain, and unless it feels very secure with your presence, it may try to escape or even bite you. Therefore, approach it slowly, talking in a reassuring tone of voice as you do so. Stoop down to the dog's level to make it even more comfortable with your presence.

You can tell a great deal about how the dog will react to you by observing its eyes and facial expression. If the dog is very submissive, it will show this by having its head slightly lowered, the mouth drawn back a little into what appears to be a smile. Occasionally a very submissive dog will even roll over on its back with the hind legs spread apart. This animal is usually easy to handle, but continue to use caution.

First, slowly attempt to pet it under the jaw. If this is accepted, then pet the top of its head while continuing to talk reassuringly. It is best not to take chances, so slip a length of rope around its neck, and then apply a muzzle. At this point, you can examine it thoroughly, and then treat the injuries.

If the dog is growling and its eyes are dilated, do not attempt to touch it. Continue to talk reassuringly, but try to slip a rope over its head and around its neck. Following this with a muzzle is necessary before you can attempt to examine it. Your goal is to ease the dog's suffering and stabilize its vital signs quickly before transporting to a veterinary surgeon.

Transporting an Injured Dog

Try not to move an injured dog more than necessary, and get it to a veterinary surgeon as soon as possible. Have someone call the veterinary surgeon to be certain he is prepared for your animal.

Depending on the injury, wrap the dog in blankets or use a blanket or flat board as a stretcher. If you suspect a broken back, a stiff board of some kind must be used. Before you move the dog, make sure the board will fit into your car. Then move it next to the dog, put the ties underneath the board, and gently lift or slide the dog onto it. Fasten the ties over the dog to eliminate as much movement as possible.

If the dog is not breathing and/or its heart is not beating, the dog will certainly die or may be dead already. CPR should be continued on the way to the veterinary surgeon. It cannot hurt and many people give up trying too early.

Animal Bite

When a dog gets into a fight with another dog, a cat, or a wild animal, damage can occur to both the skin and the underlying tissue. Many dog fights can be avoided by not permitting your dog to run loose and by keeping it on a leash when you walk it. The dog should also be trained to obey your commands.

If your dog does get into a fight, do not try to break it up with your bare hands. A fighting dog will bite anything in its way, including you. Pull your leashed dog out of harm's way or use a long stick.

When the fight is over, examine your dog carefully for hidden wounds. You'll often find punctures around the neck area and on the legs. Look through the hair carefully to find blood stains, which would indicate the skin has been punctured.

After clipping the hair from around the wound to assess the damage, flush with 3% (10 volumes) hydrogen peroxide or saline solution to prevent infection. This is one of the major complications of a bite.

The dog should then be seen by a veterinary surgeon. Although there may be only a few punctures, extensive damage may have been done to underlying muscles through the pressure of the bite. If the wounds are deep enough to require stitches, this should be done as soon as possible by a professional.

Unless there is extensive bleeding, the wounds should be left open to drain until the dog is seen by the veterinary surgeon. Whenever tissue is damaged, fluid accumulates in the area. If the wound is not left open to drain, a painful swelling will occur and the site becomes a perfect medium for the growth of bacteria and infection.

Tetanus is quite rare in dogs, but it is possible. The decision to innoculate should be left to your veterinary surgeon.

Bleeding

With a bleeding injury, the main purpose of first aid is to prevent excessive blood loss, which can lead to shock. Pressure is applied to the wound to allow the normal clotting mechanism of the blood to stop the leak. This is a complex process, but basically, the blood cells form a fine screen over the wound and thus prevent further loss of blood. That is why it is important not to remove the dressing once it has been applied. If you lift it to look at the wound, you will break up the clots that are forming and the wound will continue to bleed.

If the wound continues to bleed through the dressing, it will be necessary to use a tourniquet. The tourniquet should be used only as a last resort, because it not only stops the bleeding, it also prevents blood from getting to other tissues in the area, which become oxygen starved and die.

Blood is carried away from the heart by the arteries and returned by the veins. If an artery is cut the blood will spurt with each beat of the heart. Cut arteries require immediate care to stop the bleeding and usually require veterinary care for repair.

The paws and legs of a dog are vulnerable to injury from broken glass, nails, etc. The multiple blood vessels are close to the skin surface and are easily cut when the skin is injured. This is why the paws and legs bleed so heavily when injured.

An injured ear will also bleed heavily because the skin over the ear is so thin. A dog's reaction to an injured ear is usually to shake its head, which makes things worse. By taping the ear over the head you combat the pull of gravity and thus give the blood a better chance to clot. Firm bandaging is necessary to accomplish this.

Nails cause considerable problems to dog owners. Frequently the nails break because they get caught in ground crevices or simply break when the dog is exercising on rough ground. Clipping the nails too short is another frequent cause of bleeding. It is important to remember that nails will eventually stop bleeding if the treatment suggested in the First Aid portion of this book is followed, unless the dog has a disease which prevents clotting. In this case it should be seen at once by a veterinary surgeon.

In the centre of each nail is a blood vessel and a nerve. This is seen as the pink area in white nails, but is impossible to see on black nails, which makes them very difficult to cut. If you cut your dog's nails yourself, it is important not to cut into this "quick," as it is called, but to clip the nail just in front of it. If the "quick" is cut, the nail will bleed and the cut nerve will cause some pain. If the dog is nervous and upset, have a professional cut the nails for you. Frequent cutting will allow the blood vessel and nerve to move further back into the nail and thus allow you to cut the nail shorter.

Bloat

It is hard to accept the fact that a seemingly healthy dog can, within an hour, be fighting for its life. Bloat is an extremely serious, potentially fatal condition. Professional treatment is urgent and should not be delayed. Bloat can lead to death within a very short period of time. It seems to affect large, deep-chested dogs more than other breeds.

The symptoms are dramatic and unmistakable. The animal is usually frantically trying to vomit, but can produce nothing but thick, white mucus. The abdomen directly behind the ribs swells enormously and, when tapped with your fingers, sounds like a drum.

We have no satisfactory scientific explanation as to why bloat occurs. Basically, the stomach fills with gas, like a blown-up balloon. But with the balloon, there is room for expansion. With the stomach there is none, so the gas places pressure on the spleen, liver, and other internal organs. The result can be shock and death in a very short period of time.

We do know that excessive fermentation of food occurs in the stomach. There are apparently some toxic by-products of this fermentation that prevent release of gas build-up by the normal means of belching or passing the gas into the intestines. The bloated animal can do neither, and without immediate release of this pressure, death occurs.

Bloat is frequently followed by gastric torsion, that is, the stomach turns on itself. If this occurs, certain death will follow unless swift professional help is obtained.

To prevent bloat and subsequent torsion, feed the dog small meals several times a day rather than one large meal, and see that heavy exercise is avoided after meals.

Broken Bones

With dogs, as with human beings, all bones are subject to breakage, but leg fractures are by far the most common. It is important to remember that dogs have a high pain tolerance and often a dangling leg seems to cause no pain. Therefore, don't be afraid to handle the fractured limb (gently!). The dog will let you know if it hurts. If the dog *is* in pain or if the fracture is open, do not attempt to splint. Simply clean the wound, then hold a large towel under the limb for support and transport to a veterinary surgeon.

An open fracture is one where the bone is protruding or there is a break in the skin over the broken bone. First aid efforts should be directed to the control of infection, since the exposed bone is subject to bacterial invasion. Proper cleaning is of prime importance. Use only 3% (10 volumes) hydrogen peroxide to clean the wound. Other antiseptics may cause tissue damage.

A closed fracture is one with the bone broken but the

skin intact. The leg should be splinted, but do not confuse splinting with setting the limb, which should be done by a professional. Splinting is only a temporary procedure, so you may use any firm material at hand. The purpose of a splint is to prevent further damage by immobilizing the limb and to make the animal more comfortable during the trip to the veterinary surgeon.

Burns

Burns can be caused by fire, heat, boiling liquids, chemicals, and electricity. All are painful and can cause damage, even death. Most scalds can be avoided by care in the kitchen. Because the dog is often underfoot while its owner is cooking, care should be taken when handling hot water or cooking oil.

Superficial burns, evidenced by pain and reddening of the skin, are usually not serious. However, first aid should be given as soon as possible to ease the pain. Burns tend to "cook" the skin, and in order to stop this cooking process, cold water or ice packs should be applied to the burned area at once.

At one time the application of butter or grease was the recommended treatment, but it was discovered that these products could actually make the wound worse. They should never be used.

Third degree burns are far more serious. Depending on how much of the body is involved, they can cause death. The deeper the layers of skin involved, the more likely the dog is to go into shock. The outer skin layers are destroyed and the unprotected lower layers are then susceptible to infection. If the burns are extensive, a great deal of fluid from the tissue cells will be lost, and shock is certain to result. Therefore, treatment for shock is your first priority and should be continued until professional help can be obtained.

Chemical burns can also endanger our pets. Such products as drain cleaner or paint thinner can cause serious skin damage, and poisoning if ingested. To prevent accidents of this nature, all such products should be kept out of the dog's reach.

If you notice a chemical odour on your dog, often the first sign of this type of burn, bathe him immediately. Do not use solvents of any kind on the skin. Use mild soap and lather well; rinse thoroughly until the odour has disappeared.

Unlike heat burns, a soothing antiseptic can then be applied to the affected area until the dog can be treated by a veterinary surgeon. Be sure all the chemical is removed before the ointment is applied.

Electrical burns are most often caused by chewing on an electrical cord. The burns are almost always located on both sides of the mouth or lips. Most of these burns are minor and will heal nicely if kept clean with 3% (10 volumes) hydrogen peroxide. Electrocution is the far more serious effect of chewing on the cord. To prevent this type of injury, if you have a young puppy or if

your dog tends to chew anything in sight, do not leave it alone where cords are within its reach.

Choking

When a dog is choking on a foreign object, it needs help at once. The harder it tries to breathe, the more panicky it becomes. Your goal is to open the airway without being bitten. If you cannot reach the object with your fingers, or if the dog is struggling too much to let you try, turn it upside down and shake it. This will often dislodge the object and propel it out of the mouth.

Of course a different method must be used with a larger dog. The abdominal compression technique can be compared to pushing the air out of a beach ball. The sudden thrusts on the abdomen cause the diaphragm to bulge forward into the chest. This in turn forces air, and frequently the object, out of the windpipe.

If the dog is unconscious and you believe a foreign object is present, you must open the airway before giving artificial respiration or cardiac massage. If the dog cannot breathe, efforts to revive it will be fruitless.

The method of artificial respiration presented here is the most effective. Blowing directly into the dog's nostrils inflates the lungs to the fullest and the result is maximum oxygenation.

Cardiac massage keeps the blood pumping through the vessels and stimulates the heart muscle to contract and start beating again. With smaller dogs, you compress the heart by actually squeezing it between your hands. This keeps the blood pressure up and starts normal heart muscle contractions.

The same results are achieved with larger dogs by a different method. The chest is usually too large to compress effectively between your hands, so only one hand is used, and the chest is compressed against the floor.

The purpose of artificial respiration and cardiac massage is to keep oxygenated blood circulating to the brain. If the brain does not receive this oxygenated blood, the dog will die.

CPR (cardiopulmonary resuscitation) is a combination of artifical respiration and cardiac massage. It should be continued until the dog is breathing well by itself, or until you can get it to a veterinary surgeon. It should be continued on the way. Your continued efforts may save the dog's life.

Convulsion/ Seizure

A convulsion or seizure is rarely fatal, but it is a frightening experience when seen for the first time. It is the result of constant electrical firing of the muscles of the body from the brain.

It is important not to panic. You are not in danger, but the dog needs help to protect it from self-injury. Pull it away from walls and furniture and, if possible, wrap it in a blanket.

Do not attempt to place anything in the dog's mouth. This will not help the dog and you may be bitten. The dog is not aware of its actions during the seizure, which usually lasts only a few minutes. This is followed by 15 minutes to a half hour of recovery time, during which period the dog may be dazed and confused.

Not all seizures are due to simple epilepsy. Some are caused by lead or other poisons, liver diseases, and even brain tumours. Seizures or convulsions should never be taken lightly. The problem should be discussed with a veterinary surgeon as soon as possible.

Diarrhoea

Diarrhoea is a commonly encountered problem that occurs when food is passed through the intestine too rapidly. It can be caused by allergies, milk, worms, or spoiled food. There are also more serious causes such as tumours; viral infections; and diseases of the liver, pancreas, and kidney.

Initial home treatment should be conservative. Food should be withheld for 12 hours, but water should be available during this time as frequent diarrhoea can cause dehydration. A kaolin pectin mixture is beneficial because it coats the irritated intestinal surfaces.

The first meal should consist of a mixture of boiled minced beef or mutton, cooked rice, and cottage cheese, which is bland, easily digested and binding. This diet should be continued until stools are formed.

It is important to seek professional help if blood, severe depression, or abdominal pain are present.

Drowning

Dogs are naturally good swimmers for short distances, but they can get into trouble. Sometimes they get too far from the shore and tire trying to swim back, or fall into a swimming pool and cannot get up the steep sides.

Always protect yourself when trying to rescue a drowning dog. An extra few moments of preparation can save two lives, yours and the dog's. Once the dog is on land, you must first get the water out of its lungs. Failure to do this will certainly lead to death. Smaller dogs can simply be lifted by the hind legs, turned upside down, and shaken vigorously. A larger dog should be placed on a sloping surface with the head low and the body elevated to facilitate lung drainage.

When the lungs have been cleared, and if the dog is unconscious, it is important to check for heartbeat and breathing. If necessary, perform cardiopulmonary resuscitation (CPR). Many dogs who are seemingly dead can be revived with CPR, but if the water has not first been drained from the lungs your efforts will be useless.

Electrical Shock

Grown dogs are seldom victims of electrical shocks. But puppies are naturally curious and will chew almost anything, including electrical cords. If the insulation is punctured and the mouth comes in contact with both wires, the dog will receive a shock and may be unable to release the cord.

You must disconnect the cord from the socket immediately, before touching the dog. If you touch the dog before disconnecting the cord, you could be electrocuted.

Once the cord is disconnected you can safely touch the dog. Examine him carefully. Electrocution can cause severe heart damage and fluid accumulation in the lungs. Strong shock can stop the heart, and cardiopulmonary resuscitation (CPR) must be performed immediately to start the heart beating again.

Often the mouth will be burned from contact with the bare wires. These burns look much more serious than they are and will heal eventually if cleaned and treated properly.

Most electrical shocks require professional attention and the victim should be taken to the veterinary surgeon immediately.

Eye Injuries

Irritation of the eye can be caused by allergies, dust and dirt, lashes growing inward, fights, etc. It can result in a mild inflammation of the tissue around the eye (conjunctivitis) or severe damage to the cornea.

When examining the eye, it is important to know that dogs have a third eyelid located in the corner of the eye nearest the nose. This third eyelid can completely cover the eyeball and sometimes gives the appearance that part of the eye is gone. In addition to being a protective mechanism, it can also indicate that something is wrong with the eye. If it is raised and looks red, the eye is inflamed. Do not try to touch or manipulate this eyelid.

Other indications that the eye is irritated are squinting, and rubbing and pawing at the eye. Your first priority is to prevent self-injury since this often causes more severe damage than the original irritation.

Flat-nosed breeds with protruding eyes, such as pugs and Pekinese, are more susceptible to eye irritations than long-nosed breeds because of greater eye exposure. They are also more susceptible to having the eye actually become dislocated from its position in the skull. A "popped eye" requires immediate professional attention if it is to be saved. A clean, wet towel should be placed over the eye to keep it moist. Dehydration will certainly lead to surgical removal. The dog should then be rushed immediately to the veterinary surgeon.

Frostbite

When a dog is exposed to freezing temperatures for a long period of time, there is always the possibility of frostbite. The areas most likely to be frostbitten are those that have little or no hair and the ears and tail tip, which have a limited blood supply.

The affected areas should be warmed with moist heat, which will help to restore circulation. Frequently the skin may turn very dark, which means the tissue is dead. If this happens, see a veterinary surgeon for further treatment.

Occasionally, if damage from frostbite is severe, part of the tail or ear tips may actually fall off. Professional attention should be sought before this happens.

Heatstroke

Heatstroke is caused by the inability of the body to maintain its normal temperature because of the environmental heat. It is often caused by keeping a dog in a locked car parked in the sun, or by keeping it in any hot area without adequate ventilation.

Prompt treatment is urgent. Body temperatures often get as high as 107°F/41.5°C, and without quick cooling severe brain damage and death will occur.

Your first goal is to cool the body by immersing the dog in a cold water bath or running a garden hose on the body, either treatment to be continued for at least 30 minutes. Then apply ice packs to the head and keep them in place while transporting to a veterinary surgeon.

Heatstroke can be prevented by making sure your dog has plenty of shade and ventilation. If you must take your dog driving with you, park in the shade and leave all the windows partially open. Should heatstroke occur, prompt veterinary attention is important.

Hypothermia

Exposure to either cold water or freezing temperatures can cause hypothermia, or subnormal body temperatures. Survival will depend on how low the body temperature drops. A dog's normal body temperature is 100–101°F/38°C. If it drops below 90°F/32°C for any length of time, normal bodily functions will be severely impaired.

First aid treatment at home requires getting the dog warm again with blankets, hot water bottles or an electric blanket. Hypothermia always requires veterinary

attention as soon as initial efforts to warm the dog have been made.

Insect or Jelly-fish Sting

If the dog has been stung by a bee, wasp, or hornet, the area quickly becomes swollen and somewhat painful. The raised area is called a wheal, and if the dog has been stung more than once, you will see several of these. A possible allergic reaction to the venom deposited by the insect is the most serious problem.

If you see a wheal, apply ice to the area to reduce swelling and ease the pain. If a bee stung the dog, try to scrape the sting off with a credit card or dull knife. If it is left in the skin it will be a constant source of irritation. The bee is the only insect that will leave a sting in the skin.

If the dog has been stung by one of the insects listed above, administer a single strength cold capsule or apply antihistamine cream to the swelling. The cold capsule cannot do any harm, and since it contains an antihistamine, it may stop an allergic reaction until veterinary help is obtained.

Jelly-fish can sting a dog swimming in the sea. This should be considered if a dog shows pain or irritation after a swim and treatment carried out as for an insect sting. There may be a generalized reaction with vomiting and shivering. The vomiting is probably a mild allergic reaction and the shivering is most likely due to generalized soreness. In any event, initial treatment is the same. That is, apply ice to the area and give a cold capsule containing an antihistamine. If there is severe vomiting the cold capsule will probably not stay down. The generalized allergic reaction can lead to shock and death. Treat the victim for shock and transport immediately to the veterinary surgeon.

Poisoning

Dogs are curious creatures and like to investigate, which leads to many accidental poisonings each year. Often a dog will find an open can or bottle of some chemical and, accidentally or on purpose, spill it. Naturally the chemical gets on its fur and paws, and while licking the area clean, it swallows the possibly toxic substance. It is your responsibility as a pet owner to keep all potentially toxic products tightly closed and out of reach of your dog.

Poisoning symptoms are many and varied, as the toxic substance can be swallowed, absorbed through the skin, or inhaled. Learn to recognize the signs (listed on pages 58 and 60). It's unlikely you will be on the scene when the incident occurs.

Basic emergency treatment for different poisons is

as varied as the symptoms, so if at all possible, try to determine the poisoning agent. This is important because what is correct first aid for one is the wrong treatment for another.

For instance, if the poisoning agent is a corrosive or a petroleum product, you want to forestall vomiting since the returning chemical will cause further irritation and more severe burns. By giving olive oil or egg whites you are attempting to bind, or tie up, the chemical so it will not be absorbed.

However, if the chemical is not a corrosive or petroleum product, vomiting should be induced in order to empty the stomach of the poison. Of course it is unlikely that you will see the poison being swallowed, so in either case, professional help should be sought immediately. If the dog has vomited, the material should be taken with you to the veterinary surgeon for analysis. He will also want you to bring the suspected poison container as this will be of prime importance in determining the most effective treatment.

In addition to the obvious poisoning agents, ornamental house plants can also be dangerous to a dog. It is safe to assume that all common house plants are toxic to some degree, some more than others. When you consider that dogs often like to chew on something green, you see the problem.

The best solution is to place the plants in areas where your dog cannot reach them and use hanging baskets for the more toxic types. If in doubt, call your veterinary surgeon and tell him the type of plant you have or are going to purchase and he will tell you whether or not it poses a hazard.

Fires are another possible threat to dogs. Do not risk your own life to save your dog. Leave that task to the firefighters or those trained in rescue.

If your dog does suffer from smoke inhalation, get it away from the area and into the fresh air. If it is conscious, flush the eyes with plain water to wash out soot and other particles.

If the animal is not breathing or if the heart is not beating, use artificial respiration and/or CPR. If the smoke is intense, the airway and lungs may also be seriously damaged by inhalation of smoke and heated air. Burned lungs collect fluid, causing shortness of breath. To ease breathing, the dog's head should be kept higher than its body. Also, a burned airway may swell shut; it is imperative to keep this airway open. Immediate professional help is necessary.

Carbon monoxide poisoning can be caused by faulty heaters, but it is often due to our own carelessness. Dogs often suffer carbon monoxide poisoning from being transported in car boots. This is dangerous and inhumane.

Characteristic signs are depression, lack of coordination, heavy panting, deep red gums, and possibly convulsions. Oxygen is needed immediately and the dog should be taken to a veterinary surgeon at once. If there is no heartbeat or respiration, CPR is essential.

Puncture Wound

A puncture wound may be difficult to see because it is often covered with hair. The first sign may be a limp if it is on the leg or paw, or slightly blood-tinged fur on other parts of the body. The most common location for puncture wounds is the bottom of the paw. These wounds frequently bleed heavily because the blood vessels are so close to the surface.

If it is a body wound, you can see the extent of the injury more clearly after you have clipped the hair around the area. After cleaning the wound with 3% (10 volumes) hydrogen peroxide, examine for an imbedded foreign object, such as a splinter or shard of glass, and remove it if possible. Puncture wounds are deceptive, they can be deeper than they look. These deep wounds often damage muscle tissue, causing fluid to accumulate. It is best to leave the wound open so it can drain. This minimizes the risk of infection and swelling.

An exception to leaving the wound open would be excessive bleeding or a chest wound. Chest wounds can be very serious. If there is a hole through the entire chest wall, a "sucking" noise will be heard as the dog breathes. The act of breathing causes outside air to rush into the chest and around the lungs, causing lung collapse.

Your first priority is to seal the hole quickly to keep air from entering. If a foreign object such as a stick or an arrow is in the chest, do not attempt to pull it out. This could open the hole and lead to lung collapse. Just bandage tightly around the object and take the dog to the veterinary surgeon immediately.

Shock

Shock is extremely serious; it is the number one killer in accidents. It is a reaction to heavy internal or external bleeding or any serious injury that "scares" the body; for example, a large wound or amputation with heavy blood loss.

The body tries to compensate for the loss by speeding up the heart rate to keep the blood pressure from falling. At the same time the blood vessels that supply the outside of the body narrow. This is to conserve blood so vital organs of the body can continue to receive their normal blood supply.

However, if there is heavy blood loss or other serious injury, the body overreacts and causes a pooling of blood in the internal organs. This can cause death due to a drop in external blood pressure and possible oxygen starvation of the brain. Pale gums or cold extremities indicate shock.

When shock is present, you want to reverse the process. Elevate the hindquarters to allow more blood to reach the brain. Stop visible bleeding to prevent a drop in blood pressure. Wrap the dog in a blanket with hot water bottles to help keep the body temperature up.

This is necessary because the external blood vessels become constricted and the outside of the body becomes very cold due to lack of normal blood flow. Raising the temperature of the outside of the body helps conserve heat.

Treatment for shock cannot hurt your dog and may save its life. Shock requires professional care and the victim should be taken to the veterinary surgeon as soon as possible.

Snakebite

Poisonous snakebites are rare and the only poisonous snake in Great Britain is the adder. Snakes will not attack a dog unless provoked, but our pets are curious and bites will occur. If you live in or visit a snake area e.g. moors and heath, sunny areas or hills and woods, you can expect problems during the summer months.

If you see the dog bitten try and identify the snake. The adder has dark zigzag markings along the body and an X or Y behind the head.

If you are certain the bite was from a nonpoisonous snake, no danger really exists, except for possible infection from the bite. Since the snake mouth carries bacteria, clean the wound with 3% (10 volumes) hydrogen peroxide and use any antiseptic ointment daily.

The diagnosis of snakebite, if you did not see it happen, is based on probable exposure and symptoms the dog exhibits, listed on pages 75 and 78. Clip the hair around the suspected area to identify the type of bite. Nonpoisonous bites look like fine puncture wounds arranged in a "U" shape. If the bite has two large puncture wounds with several fine puncture wounds behind them, and the area is painful, it is probably poisonous. Immediate treatment may be needed to save the dog's life. If you are not certain whether or not the bite is poisonous, treat as poisonous.

If the dog is conscious treat for shock and keep it as quiet as possible, restricting movement to a minimum. Obtain veterinary treatment as soon as possible, and only carry out more drastic First Aid if your dog becomes unconscious or professional treatment is delayed. A tourniquet applied to a leg or tail above the bite will slow the spread of poison throughout the body. Suck the blood from the bites in order to remove as much venom as you can and thus reduce the amount of poison in the body. Use strong suction and be careful not to swallow the blood, or get bitten by your dog if it is still conscious.

After as much as possible has been sucked out, flush thoroughly by pouring 3% (10 volumes) hydrogen peroxide into the wound. The application of ice my help to reduce the spread of toxin by constricting blood vessels in the area.

Keep the tourniquet in place while transporting to the veterinary surgeon, loosening every 15 minutes for 10 seconds, then retightening. If the bite is on the face or

body, the treatment outlined above should be followed, but of course no tourniquet will be used.

The severity of the reaction caused by any poisonous snake will depend on the size of the dog and the closeness of the bite to the heart. Of course it is extremely important that treatment be started quickly after the dog has been bitten. Then immediate veterinary care is vital.

Toad Poisoning

Nature provides all life with some means of protection. Toads secrete a poisonous substance in their skin.

The poison is strong enough to cause intense irritation if it comes in contact with the mouth or eyes. The dog will salivate and may show signs of shock such as shaking head and body and a lack of co-ordination. It is important to flush the mouth or eyes immediately with copious amounts of water.

If the more serious symptoms of uncoordination or difficulty in breathing are present, contact your veterinary surgeon and start treatment for shock.

Unconsciousness

If the dog is unconscious, it is important to check its vital signs immediately. Is it breathing? Watch its chest for movement. If the dog is not breathing, artificial respiration must be performed.

Is the heart beating? If not, perform CPR (cardiopulmonary resuscitation). This is a combination of artificial respiration and cardiac massage. It may take time. It should be continued until the dog is breathing well by itself, or until you can get it to a veterinary surgeon. It should be continued on the way. Your continued efforts may save its life.

If the dog is not breathing and/or the heart is not beating, before starting treatment make sure the airway is clear. Remove any foreign material and extend the neck so he will be able to breathe. Your first priority is to get the heart beating and the dog breathing.

Watch for shock. In shock cases, the circulation to the external parts of the body is greatly diminished. Examine the gums and the inside of the upper lip. If white or very pale, shock is almost certainly present. Start treatment immediately. Shock is the number one killer in accidents.

Vomiting

Vomiting is one of the most commonly encountered problems in veterinary medicine. It is nature's way of permitting the dog to rid its stomach of an irritating substance such as spoiled food. But not all vomiting is due to simple irritation. More serious causes are viral infections or diseases of the liver, pancreas, or kidney. Initial home treatment should be conservative.

Food and water should be withheld for at least 12 hours to give the stomach time to rest and heal. Pepto-Bismol is beneficial because it coats the irritated stomach lining.

After 12 hours offer water a little at a time. Drinking too much or too fast can lead to more vomiting. The first meal should consist of a small amount of boiled minced beef or mutton, cooked rice, and cottage cheese. This is bland and easily digested. If this is held down, a transition to regular diet can be made over the next two days by mixing increasing quantities of regular dog food with the minced beef or mutton mixture.

It is important to seek professional help if there are signs of bleeding or if the dog is depressed and still vomiting after initial efforts at control have failed.

Whelping

When you first have reason to believe your bitch is pregnant, she should be given a prenatal examination by a veterinary surgeon to verify pregnancy and forestall later complications.

A dog's normal length of pregnancy (gestation period) is 61–63 days. However, delivery 1 or 2 days earlier or later is not unusual and presents no cause for alarm as long as the general health of the bitch is good.

In preparation for whelping, the bitch will make a nest with newspapers and rags if they are available. If they are not, she may dig into the carpeting with her front paws, almost as if she were digging a hole. This is termed "nest building" and is a fairly consistent sign that delivery will follow soon, usually within 2–3 days. To make your pet feel comfortable about delivering (and to save your carpet!) provide a whelping box with plenty of newspapers and rags.

One exception to this sign is a false pregnancy. If the bitch is not pregnant, but experiencing a hormonal imbalance which causes her to think she is, she will go through all the steps in preparation for delivery, even going so far as to mother a toy or other small object. As mentioned above, this is an important reason for the prenatal examination.

At about the same time the nest building occurs, you should also notice an enlargement of the breasts with milk production. Another fairly consistent method of determining when the bitch will deliver is to take her temperature each day. Approximately 24 hours before delivery, her temperature will drop about 2°F/1°C. When she is getting close to labour, a mucous discharge appears at the vulva followed by a greenish discharge. At no time should there be a brown or foul-smelling discharge. If one is present, contact your veterinary surgeon immediately.

The onset of labour will make the bitch somewhat restless, but it is not until the second stage of labour that she will actually lie down and have abdominal contractions. Once the second stage of labour begins, delivery should begin within 3 hours. If no pups are delivered by that time, professional help should be obtained.

A puppy may be born in one of three ways. The most common presentation is head and feet first. The second most common is rear legs and tail first, not to be confused with a true breech birth. In a true breech only the rump is presented, with the rear legs folded under the body of the puppy. In a small bitch, this type of presentation can cause problems and should be watched for carefully. Simple directions for assistance in delivery are listed on page 83. You will want to familiarize yourself with these procedures too, should they become necessary.

The puppies are delivered in a water-filled sac or membrane. Most bitches remove and eat this as soon as the puppy is born. However, occasionally the mother will not clean the pup, and it is up to you to do it so the pup can breathe. Clear directions are given on page 84. Familiarize yourself with them so that, if necessary, you will be prepared.

After delivery the bitch will be calm as she nurses and cleans her puppies. Don't handle the pups yourself or allow them to be handled, as this will upset the mother. The beauty of birth is a rewarding experience and many parents want their children to see it. However, they must be warned to remain still and quiet, as noise and confusion have no place during the birth process.

An injection to help evacuate the uterus of any extra material should be given by a veterinary surgeon within 24 hours after delivery.

First Aid Kit for Your Dog

Adhesive tape, 1-inch and 2-inch rolls
Gauze bandage rolls, 1-inch and 2-inch
Sterile gauze pads, 3 × 3 inches and 4 × 4 inches
Scissors
Triangular muslin bandage
2-inch and 3-inch strips of clean cloth, 2–4 feet long
Safety pins
Wooden ruler or tongue depressor for tourniquet
Wooden paint mixing sticks for splints
3% (10 volumes) hydrogen peroxide
Kaolin and pectin mixture
Pepto-Bismol
Antiseptic cream
Plastic or nylon eyedropper or dose syringe
Antihistamine cream
Single strength cold tablets or capsules
Razor blade
Ice bags (or chemical ice pack)
Empty distilled water or gallon milk containers for
   holding hot water
Blanket
Towels
4–5 feet of ¼- or ⅜-inch nylon rope for restraint
Wire cutters
Pliers
Cotton wool
Tweezers

Index

Index